Evidence-Based Approaches to Integrated Care

Edited by Mukadder Mollaoğlu, Songül Mollaoğlu, Simon George Taukeni and Murat Can Mollaoğlu

Published in London, United Kingdom

Evidence-Based Approaches to Integrated Care
http://dx.doi.org/10.5772/intechopen.1006249
Edited by Mukadder Mollaoğlu, Songül Mollaoğlu, Simon George Taukeni and Murat Can Mollaoğlu

Contributors
David Robert Matscheck, Elisabeta Shehu Kafia, Mukadder Mollaoğlu, Ingrid Flores, Irma Tchokhonelidze, Katarina Piuva, Matthew Cini, Patricia Vella Bonanno, Songül Mollaoğlu

First published in London, United Kingdom, 2025 by IntechOpen
IntechOpen is the global imprint of INTECHOPEN LIMITED, registered in England and Wales, registration number: 11086078, 167-169 Great Portland Street, London, W1W 5PF, United Kingdom

For EU product safety concerns: IN TECH d.o.o., Prolaz Marije Krucifikse Kozulić 3, 51000 Rijeka, Croatia, info@intechopen.com or visit our website at intechopen.com.

British Library Cataloguing-in-Publication Data
A catalogue record for this book is available from the British Library

Evidence-Based Approaches to Integrated Care
Edited by Mukadder Mollaoğlu, Songül Mollaoğlu, Simon George Taukeni and Murat Can Mollaoğlu
p. cm.
Print ISBN 978-1-83634-854-2
Online ISBN 978-1-83634-853-5
eBook (PDF) ISBN 978-1-83634-855-9

Meet the editors

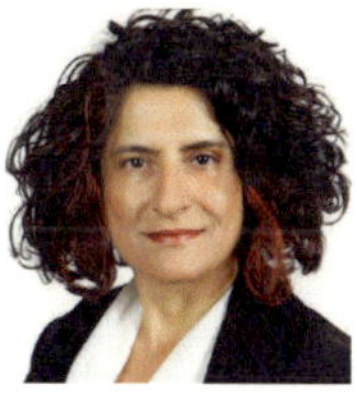

Professor Dr. Mukadder Mollaoğlu is a faculty member at the Faculty of Health Sciences, Sivas Cumhuriyet University, Turkey. Her research interests include care management in chronic diseases, quality of life, integrative therapy, and health ethics. Her research work has been published in many high-impact journals and has received numerous citations. She is an academic editor of book chapters and books. Professor Mollaoğlu received two first prizes, one in Sweden (Malmö) and the other in France (Strasbourg), for her work on life satisfaction and home care in chronic diseases. She also received the Lütfi Abay Culture and Education Foundation (LAKEV) science award in 2020 for her research in the field of health sciences.

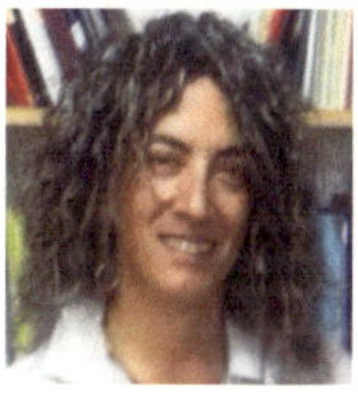

Associate Professor Dr. Songül Mollaoğlu graduated from Sivas Cumhuriyet University (SCU), Turkey, Education Faculty Fine Arts Department in 2005, and completed her master's degree in fine arts education at the Educational Sciences Institute of the same university in 2016. She completed her Ph.D. in the Fine Art Education Program at Ankara University Institute of Educational Sciences in 2021, receiving the title of Associate Professor in 2022. She has authored many articles and book chapters on art therapy and semiotics.

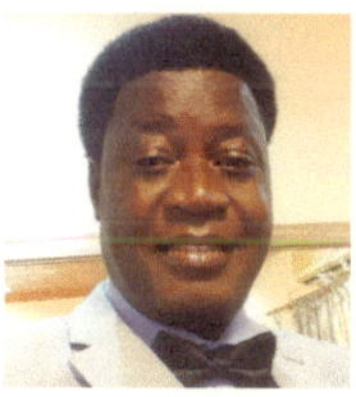

Simon George Taukeni is a professor, author, and editor working at the University of Namibia. He is a former post-doctoral research fellow at the University of Fort Hare, South Africa. Prof. Taukeni holds a Ph.D., MPH, MEd, a specialized postgraduate diploma in Behavioral and Emotional Disorder, and a BEd. He is the author of his autobiography, Against All Odds, and several edited books. Prof. Taukeni has also published numerous articles on diverse topics in health psychology, including psychosocial support, mental health, single-student mothers' dual roles, bereavement support, posttraumatic stress disorder (PTSD) among children, and more. He has collaborated with numerous local and international researchers and scholars as an editor, internal and external examiner, and principal investigator for various projects. Prof. Taukeni is one of the pioneering scientists of the biopsychosocial model of health, and he is a global citizen due to his impactful scientific contributions in Namibia, South Africa, and across the world.

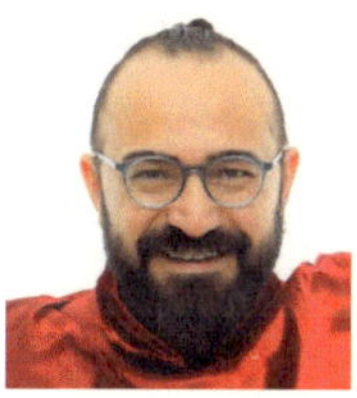

Dr. Murat Can Mollaoğlu (MD) graduated from Istanbul University Cerrahpaşa Faculty of Medicine in 2007. He became a General Surgery specialist in 2016. In 2020, he became a subspecialist in Surgical oncology. Dr. Mollaoğlu has many articles in internationally indexed journals. Dr. Mollaoğlu has treated patients with acute and chronic health problems in different health fields for many years. He has also worked as a chapter writer and book editor for many international books.

Contents

Preface

Unlike traditional treatment methods, holistic care, which utilizes care practices and approaches within healthcare systems, aims to empower individuals to take control of their environment and unleash their inner healing power. In this context, its structure, directly aligned with the philosophy of human development in healthcare, highlights the importance of holistic care practices.

Holistic care has gained extraordinary importance in the healthcare field over the last 50 years due to its close relationship with efforts to combat chronic diseases and premature death. While in the past, holistic care was considered only when other treatment options had been exhausted, today it is being used in conjunction with therapeutic approaches, starting with the diagnosis of life-threatening/terminal illnesses. Evidence-based care, a holistic process that encompasses researching the most current and advanced evidence, evaluating it with clinical expertise, and integrating research results into care practices, while also considering patient preferences, should be evident and accessible to stakeholders. This book examines the current status and developments in evidence-based integrated care approaches. It addresses a process that ensures, as with other care models, that the most current evidence supports integrated care practices, evaluates the applicability of research results, and integrates these results into the clinical arena.

In this context, this book aims to contribute to the field by bringing together current studies and information based on the need to strengthen integrated care and evidence-based approaches. We thank all the authors who contributed to the creation of this book and the staff of IntechOpen Publishing for providing us with this opportunity.

Mukadder Mollaoğlu
Faculty of Health Sciences,
Sivas Cumhuriyet University,
Sivas, Turkey

Songül Mollaoğlu
Faculty of Education,
Department of Fine Arts,
Sivas Cumhuriyet University,
Sivas, Turkey

Simon George Taukeni
University of Namibia,
Windhoek, Khomas Region, Namibia

Murat Can Mollaoğlu
VM Medical Park Maltepe Hospital,
Istanbul, Turkey

Section 1

Integrated Care

Chapter 1

Integrated Care for People with Chronic Kidney Disease

Irma Tchokhonelidze

Abstract

Chronic kidney disease (CKD) presents a significant global health challenge, affecting more than 840 million individuals and resulting in considerable morbidity, mortality, and economic strain across various healthcare systems. This chapter emphasizes the necessity for integrated care approaches that encompass early detection, effective management, and resource optimization for CKD patients. By focusing on modifiable risk factors—such as hypertension, diabetes, and obesity—the chapter underscores the importance of interdisciplinary collaboration among primary care providers, specialists, and community organizations to enhance public awareness and facilitate timely medical interventions. It also explores complications related to CKD care, such as fragmentation and polypharmacy, advocating for personalized treatment strategies tailored to individual patient circumstances. In the advanced stages of CKD, the review stresses the importance of seamless transitions to kidney replacement therapy and the incorporation of treatment options such as hemodialysis, peritoneal dialysis, kidney transplantation, and conservative care. It highlights global disparities in CKD management, particularly in low- and middle-income countries, calling for coordinated efforts, cost-effective solutions, and robust legislative frameworks to improve patient access to care. The chapter concludes that prioritizing integrated care models, addressing systemic barriers, and fostering interdisciplinary collaboration within healthcare systems can substantially improve the quality of life for CKD patients while reducing overall healthcare costs and ensuring equitable access to essential services.

Keywords: chronic kidney disease, fragmented care, interdisciplinary approach, kidney replacement therapy, integrated care

1. Introduction

Chronic kidney disease (CKD) significantly affects global mortality and morbidity, impacting countries worldwide, regardless of geographic location, income level, or healthcare infrastructure. It is estimated that over 840 million people have this progressive condition, with a prevalence rate of 8–14% [1]. In 2017, CKD resulted in 35.8 million (95% UI 33.7–38.0) disability-adjusted life years (DALYs), with diabetic nephropathy accounting for nearly one-third of these. CKD is linked to 1.4 million

 IntechOpen

(95% UI 1.2–1.6) deaths attributed to cardiovascular disease and 25.3 million (22.2–28.9) cardiovascular disease DALYs [2]. The economic burden of CKD is substantial, increasing sharply with disease severity, particularly as it progresses to kidney failure, which imposes financial strain on healthcare systems and societies. The average direct costs per patient rise sharply as CKD advances in all settings, especially upon reaching kidney failure and the initiation of kidney replacement therapy (KRT) [3]. The economic burden of diagnosed CKD and KRT is projected to grow by 9.3%. Notably, patients undergoing KRT, although only 5.3% of the diagnosed CKD population, account for 45.9% of the total costs [4]. Understanding these economic implications of CKD is crucial for allocating resources effectively and creating a sustainable healthcare system focusing on early detection and prevention of disease progression.

According to the Kidney Disease: Improving Global Outcomes (KDIGO) 2024 Clinical Practice Guideline for the Evaluation and Management of Chronic Kidney Disease, CKD is a complex condition categorized by cause (C), glomerular filtration rate (GFR) category (G1–G5), and albuminuria category (A1–A3), commonly referred to as CGA [5]. The guideline recommends incorporating clinical context, including personal and family history, social and environmental factors, medications, physical examinations, laboratory measures, imaging, and genetic and pathologic diagnosis to define the cause. The classification of CKD based on GFR and albuminuria is shown in **Table 1**.

Many underlying causes of CKD are linked to modifiable risk factors such as hypertension, atherosclerosis, cardiovascular disease, diabetes mellitus, obesity, and aging. These risk factors are widely acknowledged and largely preventable, as they contribute to other non-communicable diseases. An integrated approach involving various disciplines—including primary care physicians, endocrinologists, cardiologists, and other multidisciplinary teams—along with public awareness initiatives is vital for early detection, prompt prevention, and delay of CKD progression to kidney failure [6, 7].

The general public largely misunderstands CKD, often associating it solely with kidney failure and kidney replacement therapy rather than recognizing its prevalence

GFR stages	**GFR (mL/min/1.73 m^2)**	**Terms**
G1	≥90	Normal or high
G2	60–89	Mildly increased
G3a	45–59	Mildly to moderately decreased
G3b	30–44	Moderately to severely decreased
G4	15–29	Severely decreased
G5	<15	Kidney failure
Albuminuria stages	Albumin-to-creatinine ratio (ACR mg/g)	
A1	<300	Normal to mildly increased
A2	30–300	Mildly increased
A3	>300	Severely increased

Data from: KDIGO 2024, Clinical Practice Guideline for Evaluating and Management Chronic Kidney Disease; available at https://kdigo.org/guidelines/.

Table 1.
Chronic kidney disease (CKD) classification upon glomerular filtration rate (GFR) and albuminuria (A).

and preventability. This necessitates a public health approach that reframes CKD as a preventable chronic disease. An integrated strategy that coordinates three main domains—clinical (case and self-management), professional (multidisciplinary care team), and organizational (care programs managed by health providers)—is vital to raise awareness, with initiatives such as mass media campaigns that can enhance knowledge about CKD and encourage healthy lifestyle choices. Furthermore, this framework should prioritize early detection and preventive measures rather than allowing progression to costly interventions. Additionally, primary healthcare programs should focus on educating providers for improved early detection and management of CKD alongside the implementation of evidence-based guidelines. Advocacy is also essential, as it engages stakeholders—including health insurers and policymakers—to support CKD prevention initiatives. Plans must be tailored to consider varying levels of health literacy and cultural backgrounds to avoid exacerbating health disparities, utilizing community centers and word-of-mouth communications to reach populations with lower health literacy effectively [6].

The management of CKD people is inherently complex, necessitating an integrated strategy. The presence of multiple comorbidities in this population demands enhanced coordination of healthcare services and the development of targeted management plans for conditions such as diabetes, cardiovascular disease, hypertension, metabolic syndrome, and aging. High rates of hospitalization and mortality among CKD patients can be decreased through improved outpatient care and a focus on prevention-oriented medical practices at the level of primary care physicians [8]. The disproportionately high healthcare costs associated with the relatively small population of patients undergoing kidney replacement therapy underscore the urgent need for efficient management strategies to optimize resource allocation.

This chapter will briefly outline the role of integrated care in the early detection and progression delay of CKD and provide an overview of its significance in advanced CKD when the decision regarding kidney replacement therapy becomes essential.

2. Integrated care at the early stages of CKD

Integrating primary healthcare into the early detection of CKD is crucial for preventing kidney disease. Primary care providers (PCPs) are instrumental in the timely assessment and management of kidney patients owing to their holistic approach and frequent patient interactions [9]. PCPs play a vital role in treating modifiable risk factors for CKD, such as hypertension, cardiovascular disease, and type 2 diabetes. The asymptomatic nature of CKD often leads to delays in diagnosis, as many individuals remain unaware of their condition during the early stages due to a lack of symptoms, resulting in a considerable number of undiagnosed cases. PCPs should regularly monitor the estimated glomerular filtration rate (eGFR) and albuminuria (UACR) in at-risk populations, recommend lifestyle changes, and implement guideline-directed medical therapies, such as sodium-glucose transporter-2 (SGLT2) and renin-angiotensin-aldosterone system (RAAS) inhibitors. Treatment should be tailored to individual risk profiles, with nephrology consultations available as a part of integrated care in of rapid eGFR decline or unexplained albuminuria [10].

PCPs face several challenges, including staying current with guideline changes, managing fragmented care for CKD patients, understanding the latest treatments and their safety profiles, engaging and educating at-risk individuals, addressing the complexities of managing patients with multiple health issues, and tackling affordability and access to medications [11]. A multinational observational study found that a high percentage of patients with stage 3 CKD lacked a diagnosis code, with rates ranging from 61.6% to 95.5%. Additionally, the same study revealed concerning rates of undiagnosed conditions among patients with risk factors such as cardiovascular disease (53.0–94.4%), hypertension (59.1–94.6%), and type 2 diabetes (T2D; 50.2% to 93.7%) [12]. These challenges highlight the need for improved strategies in primary care to enhance awareness and management of CKD, aiming to improve patient outcomes through early detection and treatment. Simple actions, such as disseminating takeaways from the recently released KDIGO guideline on the Evaluation and Management of Chronic Kidney Disease (**Figure 1**), may significantly aid PCPs in early evaluations and in adopting a holistic approach to integrated care of CKD patients.

Fragmented care is often observed among individuals with diabetes mellitus, metabolic syndrome, hypertension, and obesity. This population is particularly vulnerable to cardiovascular disease (CVD) and CKD, which can adversely affect health-related quality of life and increase morbidity and mortality rates. The interconnected pathophysiological mechanisms of metabolic risk factors affecting the heart and the kidneys have been highlighted with the introduction of the cardiovascular-kidney-metabolic (CKM) syndrome by the American Heart Association. This initiative seeks to raise awareness and promote the timely prevention of CVD and CKD in at-risk people [13]. The CKM syndrome emphasizes the complexity of managing patients with these conditions, necessitating integrated care through multidisciplinary teams and healthcare systems. This integration is crucial for creating complete policies that tackle the various factors of CKM syndrome, which improves overall care plans and includes different specialties and insurance providers.

The integrated care program for CKD presents significant benefits and cost savings for patients, caregivers, and the healthcare system. Initiatives are underway to design models that integrate care for individuals with complex conditions such as diabetes and CKD. A prospective longitudinal cohort study evaluated the impact of a co-designed integrated kidney and diabetes model of care (DKS) on hospitalization rates, mortality, patient self-care, and glycemic control compared to a control group from January 2015 to October 2018. The intervention group (n = 196) demonstrated a significantly improved all-cause mortality rate (incidence rate ratio IRR 0.4 (95% CI 0.29–0.64; P < 0.0001)) compared to those who received standard care (n = 7511) [14]. Another example of the successful implementation of integrated care is a Markov model with a lifetime horizon, incorporating data from two studies: the Effectiveness of Integrated Care on Delaying Progression of Stages 3 to 4 CKD in Rural Thailand ESCORT-1 randomized control trial and the ESCORT-2 prospective cohort study, which conducts a cost-utility analysis of an integrated care program for chronic kidney disease (CKD), comparing it to conventional care. This study evaluated costs and quality-adjusted life years (QALYs) from both societal and payer perspectives, finding that the integrated care program yielded a dominant result, providing more QALYs at a lower cost than conventional care. The program was most cost-effective when implemented early in the disease progression (stages 3a and 3b) [15]. Furthermore, a randomized controlled trial in Sweden compared integrated care at a specialized clinic (intervention group) with traditional care from separate specialists (control group) involving 131 patients with diabetes, cardiovascular disease, and CKD stages 3–4. Although no significant differences were found in the major renal and cardiovascular events scores (MARCE) between the groups at the end of the study—which extended beyond 2 years for some participants—there was a notable improvement in several dimensions of health-related quality of life, including physical role, social function, and self-rated health [16].

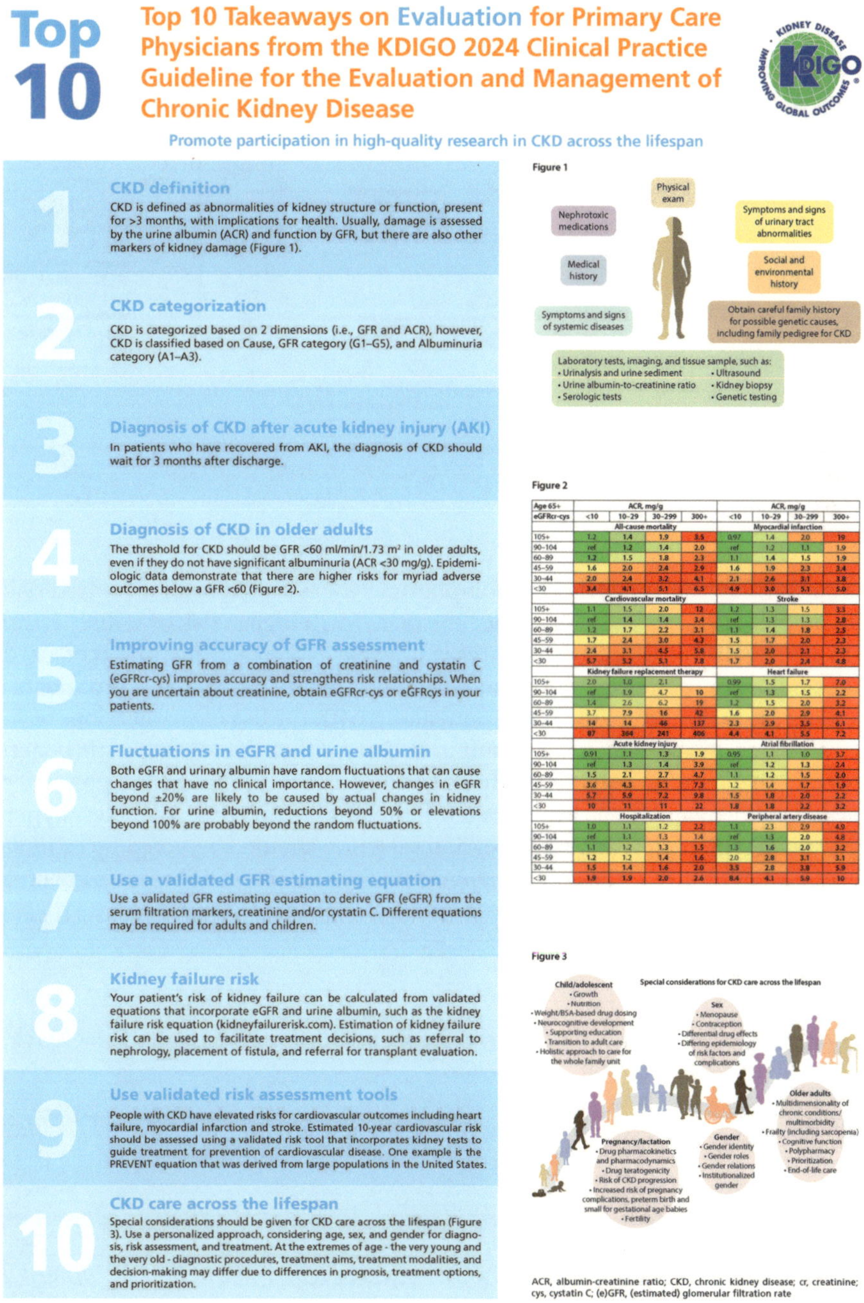

Figure 1.
Takeaway for primary care physicians from KDIGO guideline 2024 on the Evaluation and Management of Chronic Kidney Disease.

The presence of multiple comorbidities often leads to polypharmacy among these patients. Interdisciplinary collaboration in medication stewardship is essential in the CKD population. According to a systematic review by Oosting et al., over 80% of CKD patients experience polypharmacy, averaging 9.7 prescribed medications

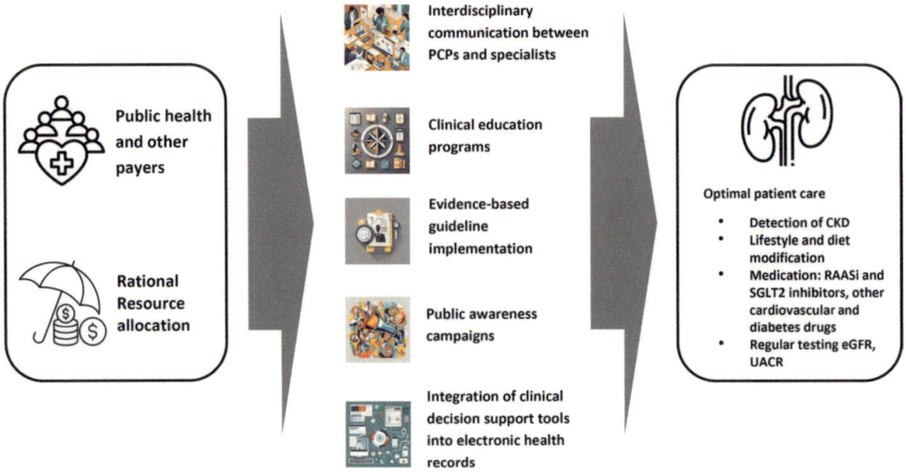

Figure 2.
Integrated care model of at early stages of CKD.

and a daily pill burden of 14.1. This polypharmacy was linked to an increased risk of all-cause mortality, a more rapid decline in eGFR, a higher risk of kidney failure, diminished quality of life, elevated rates of adverse drug reactions, and increased medication non-adherence. These issues were prevalent among all CKD patients [17]. Inaccurate estimation of kidney function, along with the use of medications with narrow therapeutic windows, can result in toxicity rather than therapeutic benefits. Reduced kidney function significantly alters the pharmacokinetics and pharmacodynamics of many medications prescribed for metabolic syndrome, diabetes, hypertension, or cardiovascular disease. Medication selection should be guided by estimated GFR (eGFR) evaluation, the risk of nephrotoxicity, regular eGFR reassessment, and dosage adjustments during acute illness [18].

2.1 Key statements

1. *Integrating primary healthcare is crucial for preventing CKD, as it allows timely detection and management by PCPs*

2. *Integrated care may lead to significant cost savings for CKD patients and healthcare systems*

3. *Integrated care improves CKD patient outcomes through early detection and treatment.*

4. *An integrative approach enhances awareness and management of CKD through collaborative care models*

Figure 2 depicts a model for integrated care in early-stage CKD.

3. Integrated care at the advanced stages of CKD

In the late stages, transitioning smoothly from progressive conditions and preparedness to kidney failure treatment can be challenging. Integrated kidney care focuses on a sustainable approach to enhancing the health of individuals with kidney failure, considering local factors and societal preferences. The model should integrate various treatment options, such as hemodialysis (HD), peritoneal dialysis (PD), kidney transplantation, conservative management, and connections among these modalities. The best model aims to benefit patients, families, communities, and healthcare systems. Logistical, social, and ethical considerations must be addressed to maximize benefits from any modality. PD is often recommended over HD due to its cost-effectiveness, scalability, and suitability for remote areas [19].

However, higher initial costs in some regions sometimes hinder public funding for PD. Addressing this involves local manufacturing, reimbursement reforms, and training medical staff. Kidney transplantation is the optimal option for appropriate patients, offering better survival rates and a higher quality of life at lower costs. However, the promotion of preemptive kidney transplantation and home dialysis is often insufficient, leading to unnecessary costs and compromised patient care [19, 20].

Global variations in kidney failure care exist. Significant heterogeneity is present in investment levels for preventing, diagnosing, and treating kidney disease, influenced by health systems, values, resources, and competing interests. Currently, kidney failure care remains fragmented in many countries, leading to missed opportunities for improved patient experiences, better population health, and cost reduction. Several models of integrated kidney care are discussed in the United States, including ESRD Seamless Care Organizations (ESCOs), programs under the proposed Dialysis Patients Act, and the Renal Physicians Association Incident ESRD Clinical Episode Payment Model (RPA Model) [21]. These models all aim to promote home dialysis, each with advantages and disadvantages. The ESCO model is highlighted for its successful track record, but concerns are raised about its scalability and potential to consolidate care among larger organizations. The Dialysis Patients Act is not entirely provider-neutral and could be detrimental to smaller organizations and patient choice. All models require revision to address access to transplantation better, incentivize timely dialysis when appropriate, improve advance care planning, and prioritize patient well-being over financial concerns [22]. Principles for Integrated Nephrology Care Delivery Models proposed by the American Society of Nephrology (ASN) are summarized in **Table 2**.

According to a systematic review by Nkunu et al., CKD care models in LMICs differ in service provision [23]. While some models provide comprehensive care, others focus on fragmented care, primarily emphasizing early-stage prevention. Nevertheless, most models incorporate key elements such as the management of cardiovascular disease, diabetes, and blood pressure. Additionally, interdisciplinary care teams are present in most models, particularly during the preparation for kidney replacement therapies [24]. However, conservative management remains underrepresented. Access to transplant workups often necessitates referrals to larger centers, which can create barriers for patients [25].

The framework for establishing integrated care programs in low- and middle-income countries (LMICs) poses a significant challenge due to the high cost of treatment. An integrated approach, combining conservative management, transplantation and dialysis, is crucial for sustainability and better patient outcomes. This approach considers resource use and prioritizes interventions based on cost-effectiveness. When kidney replacement therapy is necessary, transplantation offers the best outcomes at a lower cost. PD is suggested as a cost-effective alternative to HD in resource-constrained settings, especially in remote areas. The need for coordination

Key principals of integrated care model for chronic kidney disease	Explanation
Comprehensive patient care	Integrated models should encompass the full spectrum of kidney disease, from late-stage CKD to kidney failure including dialysis, transplantation, and palliative care. This approach aims to improve care coordination, reduce fragmentation, and optimize cost savings. Including late-stage CKD patients helps mitigate the risk of selecting only the most financially rewarding patients.
Diversity of dialysis providers	The models should involve a diverse range of dialysis provider sizes and types to foster innovation and ensure patient choice. Maintaining this diversity is especially crucial considering the market share held by a small number of large providers.
Promoting preemptive transplants	Models must actively promote preemptive kidney transplantation as the optimal treatment for suitable ESRD patients. This includes encouraging living donor transplants and facilitating access to transplant services.
Nephrologist leadership	Nephrologists should maintain a leadership role in the design and implementation of these models due to their comprehensive understanding of kidney patient care across all stages of the disease. Their involvement ensures the models prioritize patient well-being and cost-effectiveness.
Facilitating research and innovation	The models should generate data accessible to the research community, fostering innovation in both kidney failure without and with dialysis care. This addresses the current lack of substantial research and development investment in the dialysis industry.
Safeguards against preferential patient selection	Mechanisms should be in place to monitor and prevent the selection of only the most profitable patients and to ensure equitable access to care and consistent outcomes. This is particularly important given the potential for incentives to skew patient selection.

Key principals based on analysis of the document "ASN Principles for Integrated Nephrology Care Delivery Models," available at www.asn-online.

Table 2.
Principles for Integrated Nephrology Care Delivery Models proposed by the American Society of Nephrology (ASN).

among different healthcare components, international collaboration, and partnerships is essential to ensure a sustainable and equitable system for managing kidney failure in LMICs [26].

Prerequisites for establishing a national kidney transplant program are: (1) effective legislation for protecting organ donors and recipients and preventing organ trafficking; (2) multidisciplinary team expertise across various specialties (surgery, nephrology, infectious disease, etc.); (3) infrastructure for adequate facilities, including immunology laboratories and supportive dialysis services; (4) national registries for data collection, tracking outcomes, and ensuring quality; (5) community engagement for public education and supporting organ donation; (6) financial sustainability mechanisms to cover the organizational, interventional, and long-term immunosuppressive treatment [20, 24].

The International Society of Nephrology has developed a strategic plan to enhance global access to safe, sustainable, and equitable integrated care for patients with kidney failure. This plan includes establishing robust data collection and monitoring systems to track progress and inform decision-making, utilizing renal registries and resources like the ISN Global Kidney Health Atlas (ISN-GKHA). It outlines: (1) defining safe minimum standards for dialysis, developing quality frameworks, establishing training and support infrastructures, and addressing barriers to implementation,

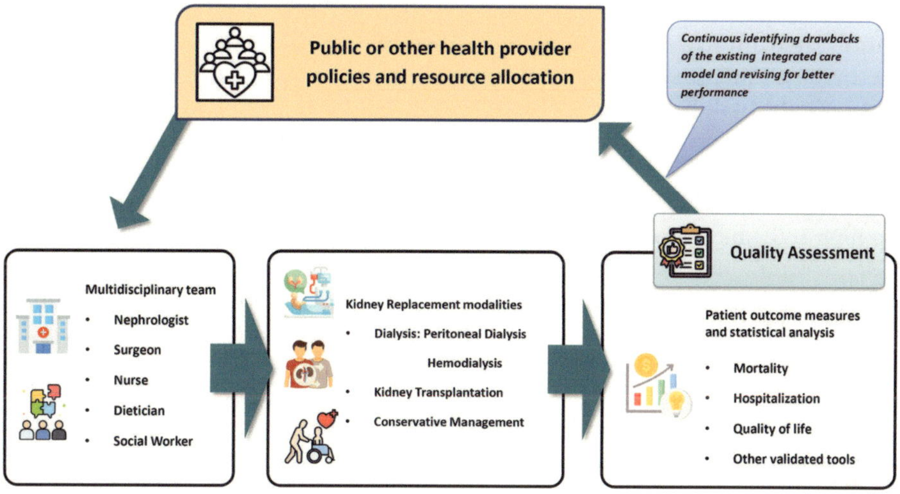

Figure 3.
Integrated care model of patients with kidney failure.

such as governance issues, resource limitations, and workforce shortages; (2) identifying essential workforce competencies, developing training programs, and assessing resource needs beyond the workforce (such as infrastructure and funding); (3) creating assessment tools for transplant readiness, reviewing existing transplant programs, and supporting their development; (4) supporting the creation of conservative care programs in areas where they do not exist. The plan advocates for a multifaceted approach involving patients, governments, healthcare institutions, industry, and researchers to create action plans and deliverables for each theme, emphasizing the need for collaboration, data-driven decision-making, and the ability to adapt strategies to various resource settings [27]. **Figure 3** depicts the integrated care model in kidney failure.

3.1 Key statements

1. *Integrated kidney care emphasizes a sustainable approach for individuals with kidney failure, incorporating various treatment options and considering local factors and societal preferences*

2. *Many countries have fragmented kidney failure care, leading to missed opportunities for improved patient experiences and population health outcomes*

3. *Integrated care interlinks treatment options, such as hemodialysis, peritoneal dialysis, kidney transplantation, and conservative care, for effective patient care*

4. *Significant heterogeneity exists in kidney failure care investment and approaches, influenced by varying health systems, values, resources, and competing interests*

5. *Integrated care of kidney failure advocates for a collaborative, data-driven approach involving governments, healthcare institutions, industry, patients, and researchers to address kidney care challenges globally*

In conclusion, addressing chronic kidney disease (CKD) requires a comprehensive and integrated approach encompassing all disease stages, including kidney replacement therapy. The considerable global burden of CKD, exacerbated by its association with modifiable risk factors and increasing treatment costs, underscores the urgency of implementing effective early detection and management strategies. Integrated care models that involve multidisciplinary teams are essential for optimizing patient outcomes, particularly in populations with multiple comorbidities. Increased public awareness and education can bridge the knowledge gap regarding the preventability of CKD, encouraging healthier lifestyle choices and timely medical intervention.

Moreover, establishing structured care programs in both high- and low-income settings is vital to ensure equitable access to essential services such as transplantation and dialysis. In lower-income countries, focusing on cost-effective solutions like peritoneal dialysis and a strong legislative framework for organ donation could greatly enhance patient care and outcomes. Moving forward, fostering collaboration among healthcare providers, policymakers, and communities is essential to creating sustainable and efficient health systems that respond to the needs of CKD patients.

Ultimately, by prioritizing integrated care, promoting interdisciplinary collaboration, and addressing systemic barriers, we can significantly improve the quality of life for individuals with CKD, reduce the economic burden on healthcare systems, and ensure that all patients receive the timely, compassionate, and high-quality care they deserve.

Author details

Irma Tchokhonelidze[1,2]

1 Tbilisi State Medical University, Tbilisi, Georgia

2 Tbilisi State Medical University and Ingorokva High Medical Technology University Clinic, Tbilisi, Georgia

*Address all correspondence to: i.tchokhonelidze@tsmu.edu

References

[1] Kovesdy CP. Epidemiology of chronic kidney disease: An update 2022. Kidney International. Supplement (2011). 2022;**12**(1):7-11. DOI: 10.1016/j.kisu.2021.11.003

[2] GBD Chronic Kidney Disease Collaboration. Global, regional, and national burden of chronic kidney disease, 1990-2017: A systematic analysis for the Global Burden of Disease Study 2017. Lancet. 2020;**395**(10225):709-733. DOI: 10.1016/S0140-6736(20)30045-3

[3] Jha V, Al-Ghamdi SMG, Li G, Wu MS, Stafylas P, Retat L, et al. Global economic burden associated with chronic kidney disease: A pragmatic review of medical costs for the inside CKD research programme. Advances in Therapy. 2023;**40**(10):4405-4420. DOI: 10.1007/s12325-023-02608-9. Epub 2023 Jul 26

[4] Chadban S, Arıcı M, Power A, Wu MS, Mennini FS, Arango Álvarez JJ, et al. Projecting the economic burden of chronic kidney disease at the patient level (*Inside CKD*): A microsimulation modelling study. EClinicalMedicine. 2024;**72**:102615. DOI: 10.1016/j.eclinm.2024.102615

[5] Kidney Disease: Improving Global Outcomes (KDIGO) CKD Work Group. KDIGO 2024 Clinical practice guideline for the evaluation and management of chronic kidney disease. Kidney International. 2024;**105**(4S):S117-S314

[6] Dorgelo A, Oostrom TAJ. An integrated approach towards a public health perspective on chronic kidney disease. Nature Reviews. Nephrology. 2022;**18**(3):131-132. DOI: 10.1038/s41581-022-00537-4

[7] Li PK, Garcia-Garcia G, Lui SF, Andreoli S, Fung WW, Hradsky A, et al. Kidney health for everyone everywhere—From prevention to detection and equitable access to care. Clinical Nephrology. 2020;**93**(3):111-122. DOI: 10.5414/CNWKDEditorial

[8] Valentijn PP, Schepman SM, Opheij W, Bruijnzeels MA. Understanding integrated care: A comprehensive conceptual framework based on the integrative functions of primary care. International Journal of Integrated Care. 2013;**13**:e010. DOI: 10.5334/ijic.886

[9] Neale EP, Middleton J, Lambert K. Barriers and enablers to detection and management of chronic kidney disease in primary healthcare: A systematic review. BMC Nephrology. 2020;**21**(1):83. DOI: 10.1186/s12882-020-01731-x

[10] Kushner P, Khunti K, Cebrián A, Deed G. Early identification and management of chronic kidney disease: A narrative review of the crucial role of primary care practitioners. Advances in Therapy. 2024;**41**(10):3757-3770. DOI: 10.1007/s12325-024-02957-z. Epub 2024 Aug 20

[11] Nee R, Yuan CM, Narva AS, Yan G, Norris KC. Overcoming barriers to implementing new guideline-directed therapies for chronic kidney disease. Nephrology, Dialysis, Transplantation. 2023;**38**(3):532-541. DOI: 10.1093/ndt/gfac283

[12] Tangri N, Moriyama T, Schneider MP, Virgitti JB, De Nicola L, Arnold M, et al. Prevalence of undiagnosed stage 3 chronic kidney disease in France, Germany, Italy, Japan and the USA: Results from the multinational observational REVEAL-CKD study. BMJ Open.

2023;**13**(5):e067386. DOI: 10.1136/bmjopen-2022-067386

[13] Ndumele CE, Rangaswami J, Chow SL, Neeland IJ, Tuttle KR, Khan SS, et al. Cardiovascular-kidney-metabolic health: A presidential advisory from the American Heart Association. Circulation. 2023;**148**(20):1606-1635. DOI: 10.1161/CIR.0000000000001184

[14] Zimbudzi E, Lo C, Ranasinha S, Earnest A, Teede H, Usherwood T, et al. A co-designed integrated kidney and diabetes model of care improves mortality, glycaemic control and self-care. Nephrology, Dialysis, Transplantation. 2022;**37**(8):1472-1481. DOI: 10.1093/ndt/gfab230

[15] Paffett M, Phannajit J, Chavarina KK, Chuanchaiyakul T, Jiamjariyapon T, Thanachayanont T, et al. Economic evaluation of an integrated care program compared to conventional care for patients with chronic kidney disease in rural communities of Thailand. Kidney International Reports. 2024;**9**(8):2546-2558. DOI: 10.1016/j.ekir.2024.05.012

[16] Evén G, Stenfors T, Jacobson SH, Jernberg T, Franzén-Dahlin Å, Jäghult S, et al. Integrated, person-centred care for patients with complex cardiovascular disease, diabetes mellitus and chronic kidney disease: A randomized trial. Clinical Kidney Journal. 2024;**17**(11):sfae331. DOI: 10.1093/ckj/sfae331

[17] Oosting IJ, Colombijn JMT, Kaasenbrood L, Liabeuf S, Laville SM, Hooft L, et al. Polypharmacy in patients with CKD: A systematic review and meta-analysis. Kidney360. 2024;**5**(6):841-850. DOI: 10.34067/KID.0000000000000447. Epub 2024 Apr 25

[18] Hall RK, Kazancıoğlu R, Thanachayanont T, Wong G, Sabanayagam D, Battistella M, et al. Drug stewardship in chronic kidney disease to achieve effective and safe medication use. Nature Reviews. Nephrology. 2024;**20**(6):386-401. DOI: 10.1038/s41581-024-00823-3. Epub 2024 Mar 15

[19] DCH H, Davies SJ, Finkelstein FO, Jha V, Bello AK, Brown M, et al. Strategic plan for integrated care of patients with kidney failure. Kidney International. 2020;**98**(5S):S117-S134. DOI: 10.1016/j.kint.2020.07.023

[20] O'Connell PJ, Brown M, Chan TM, Claure-Del Granado R, Davies SJ, Eiam-Ong S, et al. The role of kidney transplantation as a component of integrated care for chronic kidney disease. Kidney International. Supplement (2011). 2020;**10**(1):e78-e85. DOI: 10.1016/j.kisu.2019.11.006. Epub 2020 Feb 19

[21] Brady BM, Erickson KF. Integrated care in ESKD: A perspective of nephrologists. Clinical Journal of the American Society of Nephrology. 2019;**14**(3):451-453. DOI: 10.2215/CJN.13081118. Epub 2019 Jan 29

[22] Johnson DS, Meyer KB. Integrated care for people with kidney disease: The perspective of a nonprofit dialysis provider. Clinical Journal of the American Society of Nephrology. 2019;**14**(3):448-450. DOI: 10.2215/CJN.13641118

[23] Nkunu V, Wiebe N, Bello A, Campbell S, Tannor E, Varghese C, et al. Update on existing care models for chronic kidney disease in low- and middle-income countries: A systematic review. Canadian Journal of Kidney Health and Disease. 2022;**9**:20543581221077505. DOI: 10.1177/20543581221077505

[24] Collister D, Pyne L, Cunningham J, Donald M, Molnar A, Beaulieu M, et al. Multidisciplinary chronic kidney disease clinic practices: A scoping review. Canadian Journal of Kidney Health and Disease. 2019;**6**:2054358119882667. DOI: 10.1177/2054358119882667

[25] Davison SN, Pommer W, Brown MA, Douglas CA, Gelfand SL, Gueco IP, et al. Conservative kidney management and kidney supportive care: Core components of integrated care for people with kidney failure. Kidney International. 2024;**105**(1):35-45. DOI: 10.1016/j.kint.2023.10.001

[26] Tonelli M, Nkunu V, Varghese C, Abu-Alfa AK, Alrukhaimi MN, Fox L, et al. Framework for establishing integrated kidney care programs in low- and middle-income countries. Kidney International Supplements (2011). 2020;**10**(1):e19-e23. DOI: 10.1016/j.kisu.2019.11.002. Epub 2020 Feb 19. Erratum in: Kidney Int Suppl (2011). 2020; 10(2):e186. DOI: 10.1016/j.kisu.2020.11.001

[27] ISN-Global Kidney Health Atlas. Available from: https://www.theisn.org/initiatives/global-kidney-health-atlas/

Chapter 2

Coordinated Individual Planning for Complex Needs with Service User Involvement in Sweden: A Question of Collaboration Competence?

David Robert Matscheck and Katarina Piuva

Abstract

Sweden has a reputation for having one of the most advanced welfare states in the world, but has problems with fragmentation of care, caused by specialization and exacerbated by the increasing domination of organizational steering by principles of New Public Management (NPM). People with concomitant mental health and substance abuse problems are one group which is affected, as these individuals often have complex needs involving health and social care from specialized competences in different sectors and organizations. In Sweden, as in other countries, there has been limited impact for collaborative models intended to address the problem of fragmentation of care, such as case management and team-based models such as ACT and FACT. In 2009, the coordinated individual plan (CIP) was introduced in an attempt to scale up collaboration for these individuals and other target groups. CIP is also presented as a tool for increasing service users'/patients' involvement in their own care. A research project including two studies of case files and an interview study has found that impact has been limited. Neo-institutional theory and theories of street-level bureaucracy in the context of NPM suggest a need for greater "collaboration competence" across organizations and professions.

Keywords: case coordination, individual plans, complex needs, collaboration, service user involvement, collaboration competence

1. Introduction

> *In practice, collaboration is impossible to achieve when it is most important. Calls for collaboration are heard when help and interventions are needed which lie outside the specialized competence of the respective collaboration partners. Collaboration is expected to happen in a no-man's land where the professionals involved have no common base of knowledge.*
>
> *Börjeson (author's translation) [1]*

Sweden has long had a reputation for having one of the most advanced welfare states in the world. Especially since the second World War, universal health and economic benefits have been combined with specialized forms of care and social interventions for children and families, people with chronic illnesses and disabilities, and elderly. The Health and Medical Services Act of 1982 [2] and the Social Service Act of 1980 [3] provided the legislative base for the system which, in its essential structure, still applies today, featuring a healthcare sector and a separate social care sector. Both were and still are publicly financed and were originally operated by local and regional authorities belonging to the state.

With time, specialization, which has become more and more developed following scientific advances in many areas of medical health care, has spread to social care. While the Social Service Act in its original version from 1980 emphasized a holistic approach, social care interventions have tended to be more and more focused on specific kinds of problems, and social workers have been encouraged to develop competence in these specific areas. In both sectors, the tendency has been to increasing fragmentation of care [4–6].

The development of the welfare state was made possible in large part by the extended period of economic growth which followed World War II. But by the 1980s growth had begun to slow, eventually leading to a crisis in public finances in the beginning of the 1990s. At the same time, there was growing criticism of the bureaucratic systems of administrating public services, focusing on claims of inefficiency and lack of choice for individual patients and service users [7].

In this climate, and in a development parallel to that in other European countries, ideas and principles belonging to New Public Management (NPM) were introduced. NPM has since come to dominate public institutions in Sweden, not least in the health and social care sectors. NPM prioritizes economic efficiency achieved by principles from the private sector including business, competition, and quantifiable measures of effectiveness. These principles can come in conflict with already existing principles based on laws and regulations, public financing, and professional ethics [7–10].

The above quote, from the late Swedish nestor and the first Professor in Social Work at Stockholm University Bengt Börjeson, expresses the problem which has bedeviled the welfare state from the start, not least in the areas of health and social care. Many conditions and problems are not easily categorized or involve different perspectives which are dependent one another. As Professor Börjeson remarked, the various professionals lack a common base of knowledge and perspective. They also come from different organizational environments based on different economic and legal requirements. The increasing dominance of NPM has exacerbated these problems, placing emphasis on each organization's and department's interest in economic efficiency, instead of on the best interests of the patient/service user. It is in this environment that calls have come for greater and better collaboration and integrated care.

The authors' focus has been on people with concomitant mental health and substance abuse problems. These individuals often have a wide variety of medical and social issues and can be characterized as having complex needs. Meeting these needs can involve specialized medical and psychiatric care, psychosocial interventions, help with personal economy, work-related rehabilitation, and more requiring specialized professionals with various competences and in different sectors and organizations. Integrated care and collaboration have for many years been recognized as necessary areas of development to meet the challenges of care for this group [11].

In the chapter, we will summarize the different approaches which have been attempted, eventually leading to the main focus of our research in this area, the coordinated individual plan (CIP). We conclude that, for initiatives for improved collaboration to be successful, there is a need not only for organizational tools such as CIP, case management, or multidisciplinary teams, but for a general increased level of "collaboration competence" among professionals in the care sectors.

2. Care for complex needs in Sweden

Sweden, along with the other Nordic countries, was one of the last countries in Europe to deinstitutionalize psychiatric care [12]. When the Swedish Mental Health Care Reform was finally implemented in 1995, following a parliamentary decision in 1994 [13, 14], the responsibility for care was divided between welfare organizations in a way that required in-depth collaboration. Social services in the local authorities were given responsibility for housing, employment, and daily activities, while the regional medical care system was given continued responsibility for psychiatric care. The justification for the reform was twofold. Humanitarian and economic motives coincided with arguments for a deinstitutionalization of mental healthcare. On the one hand, the reform was justified as a normalization of life for the mentally ill. On the other hand, the economic crisis in the 1990s facilitated the parliamentary decision to reduce the number of medical hospital beds. The institutions for the mentally disabled, which were very expensive to run, had already been closed and replaced by community care [13, 14].

This reduction of hospital care was the final step in an ongoing organizational change from medical responsibility governed by the regions toward community care governed by local authorities. However, the group of individuals with complex needs due to concomittant substance abuse problems and mental illness was underrepresented in the problem description behind the Swedish Mental Health Care Reform. The result was a triple fragmentation of care for individuals with complex needs: (1) In terms of organizational borders between medical care under the county councils, and social care, including daily living and housing, under municipal local authorities, (2) in terms of an internal division of medical responsibility, the borders between psychiatric care and medical care of substance addiction, and (3) care of individuals with substance abuse is also a responsibility of the local authorities, who provide addiction treatment through the procurement of private healthcare providers. To summarize, we can conclude that care of these patients is affected both by internal boundaries within the welfare organizations and by boundaries between the administrations of medical care and community care [13, 15, 16].

The dominance of NPM is another factor which has impeded the opportunities for adequate care for individuals with complex needs. One feature of NPM which has had a particularly large impact in the care sectors is the purchaser-provider split [9, 10, 13]. That is, the division of responsibilities between organizational departments for budgeting and ordering services, and the operative organizations which are to provide the actual care to patients and service users. Ordering of services remains the responsibility of the local and regional authorities, but operations are now in a mix of private and public organizations according to market-based principles. In the social service, services are ordered on the individual level by departments for needs assessment and carried out by providers which sometimes are in the private sector, exacerbating fragmentation of care. In addition, restrained use of public funds and performance-oriented short-term goals do not favor forms of care which require longer processes in contact with patients/service users, as are often necessary in working with these individuals.

It is within this context that the Swedish state has attempted to encourage greater use of collaborative forms for integrated care. National guidelines and recommendations have been developed and circulated, citing evidence for the effectiveness of forms such as case management, multidisciplinary "ACT-teams" (Assertive Community Treatment), and co-location. Economic stimulants have also been used, with state support granted to projects for implementation of these and other evidence-based forms and models [17].

Even in theory, case management and multidisciplinary team forms such as ACT or Flexible Assertive Community Treatment (FACT) can only reach small numbers of patient/service users, since the basic principle is to focus specialized resources on the individuals who have the greatest need. Nevertheless, it has proved difficult both to build teams, especially across the two main organizational sectors, and to sustain those teams which have eventually started [17]. Co-location had some initial success but has also been difficult to sustain. On the whole, success has been limited for all of these forms.

Partly in response to this situation, there has been an ambition to reach larger numbers of individuals in a kind of scaling up of coordinated care. Norway's individual care plan (ICP), which was legislated in 2001, helped serve as an inspiration. The goal of the ICP is to counter fragmentation, but also to increase user involvement. An ICP is mandatory whenever a patient/service user desires one. It features a care plan with a trained coordinator and interprofessional "responsibility groups" around the individual [18]. The ICP has had some success but appears to have been used less than was hoped for. CIP can also be compared to the care program approach (CPA) in England and Wales, which has been met with skepticism from both professionals and service user/patients [19]. A more recent version of these ideas is the Community Health Framework, which has been introduced in an attempt to make the CPA more flexible and responsive to individual needs [20].

Sweden's answer to the challenge of scaling up integrated care came in 2009, when legislation was passed requiring coordinated individual plans (CIP) and local collaboration agreements [21]. A CIP is mandatory when coordinated planning is judged to be necessary either by health care or by the social service. This model is an attempt to reach more users/patients by making collaboration mandatory for all professionals in both sectors, rather than reaching only those who are served by collaboration teams in places where recommended models have been implemented. Like the ICP, CIP is presented as a tool for increasing users'/patients' involvement in their own care, with voluntary participation and requiring the individual's consent [22].

3. CIP: An overview of the research

A CIP is started when a professional within either a healthcare unit or a social service unit calls a CIP meeting. Patients/service users cannot call CIP meetings themselves, but guidelines stipulate that a CIP should be called if the patient/service user wishes. A CIP requires the patient/service user's consent but is only a plan and there is no formal recourse, neither for the patient/service user nor for any other part if the proposed treatments or interventions do not take place [23].

A basic feature of CIP is that it involves a wide range of services and organizations. In addition to the health and social sectors, the state's employment service, social insurance, and correctional services can be involved (**Figure 1**). This means that a CIP can have as few as two or three participants (in addition to the patient/service user), or as many as nine or ten.

Neither the law nor any guidelines stipulate a specific coordinator for a CIP. Usually, the professional who has called the CIP meeting also leads the meeting and is responsible for documentation. Professionals with experience of CIP describe a meeting process which begins with asking the patient/service user their view of their needs and then going around the circle, with each professional giving their view and what they can offer. The CIP document must be signed by all the units who are represented, as well as by the patient/service user [23].

The authors' research project constitutes a large part of the existing research on CIP, particularly concerning adults with complex needs. The project included two case file studies and an interview study which have been published in four articles [23, 25–27]. A project with a similar focus was started a few years later by Ulla-Karin Schön and colleagues [28]. A study of CIP and an overlapping group, adults with disabilities, has also been published [29], and there is also an earlier study of CIP and young people [30].

3.1 Two file studies on CIP: An uneven model with a low level of collaboration

The authors' project was conducted in the Stockholm region, using data collected from social service units in local authorities and interviews with professionals in local authorities and their collaborative partners in mental health and substance abuse

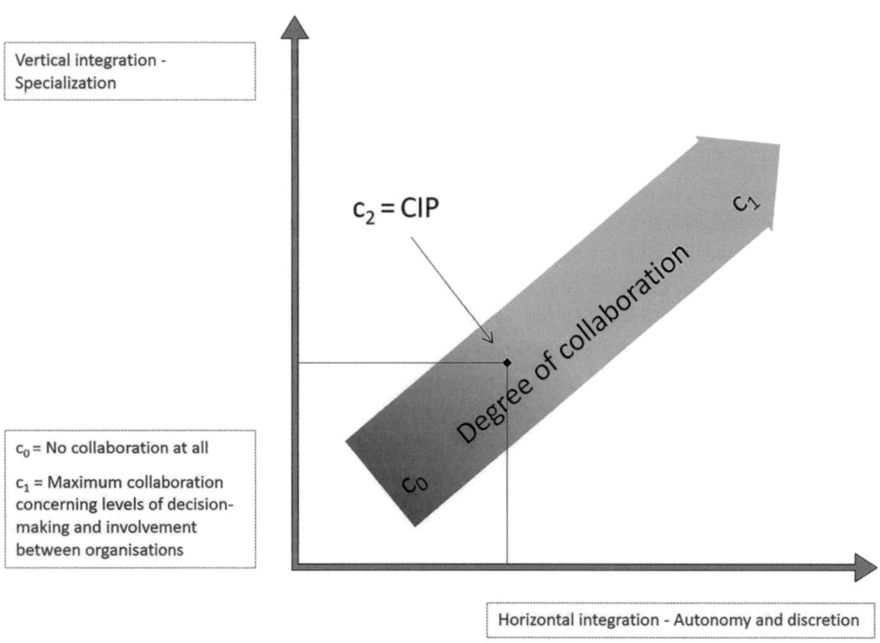

Figure 1.
Model for analysis of collaboration structure as adapted from Axelsson and Bihari-Axelsson [24], and degree of collaboration indicated by CIP documents and other case documentation [23, 25].

treatment in the regional healthcare system. Stockholm is the most populous region in Sweden, with a total population of about 2.3 million, which allowed for the selection of relatively comprehensive data. Our studies were conducted in the local authorities in the northeastern and northwestern areas in the region. Quantitative data has been compiled, presenting an overview of in what ways CIP has been used, and complemented with qualitative data for deeper understanding of CIP as a phenomenon. In the resulting analyses, we have used three different theoretical perspectives which in turn complement each other for the comprehensive analysis which we will present in our final discussion.

In the case file studies, social service files from units for substance abuse and mental health were selected in which at least one CIP had been done during the years 2014–2016. In the first study [23], two files were selected from each of six local authorities. In the second study [25], all files with CIP in one local authority were studied, a total of 25 files. Data was extracted using a protocol including demographic data, substance abuse and mental health problems, physical health, social problems, and other circumstances. Data was also compiled concerning who had initiated the CIP, which professionals and organizations were represented, how the individual's needs were formulated, and what actions and interventions were agreed upon, and what treatments and interventions had taken place and been followed up. Finally, data was extracted concerning service user/patient involvement in CIP. In addition, we studied local collaboration agreements in the local authorities for an analysis of organizational supporting structures for CIP.

In both case file studies, Axelsson and Bihari Axelsson's conceptual framework was used for the theoretical analysis [24]. This framework is in turn based on contingency theory as presented by Lawrence and Lorsch [31]. The framework includes a "conceptual scheme" involving a vertical axel, which represents the organizational hierarchy, and a horizontal axel, which represents contacts among units in the different organizations. In our analysis, we have modified the model so that the vertical axel also represents the tendency to specialization, while the horizontal axel represents the degree of autonomy and possibilities for discretion for professionals. We have also included user participation on the horizontal axel. We have then used the modified model to evaluate the degree of collaboration achieved by using this modified model (**Figure 1**).

A consequence of contingency theory is that, in a situation in which there is a high degree of organizational differentiation, a complex model is needed to achieve a high degree of collaboration [24]. We have used a scale developed by Andersson et al. which places simple collaborative models such as information exchange, case coordination, and interagency meetings at the low end of the scale, team models such as case management and ACT toward the middle, and more complex models such as co-location and pool budgets at the high end [32]. In our analysis, we have attempted to place CIP within this scale, to judge whether CIP is adequate to meet the need for collaboration around the target groups.

3.1.1 Findings from the file studies

When selecting files for the first file study, it immediately became obvious that CIP was used very unevenly in the different local authorities. Two local authorities did not participate in the study because they had no CIPs at all for the target groups or had no efficient way of finding which files had CIPs. The other local authorities varied between 2 and 33 files for the authors to select from [23].

Our first finding was that CIPs were called equally often by healthcare professional, either in substance abuse/addiction treatment or in social psychiatric care, as by a social service unit, usually by a professional for needs assessment (in Sweden these are called "social secretaries," sometimes translated as "social welfare secretaries") but sometimes by a social care provider. The CIP was seldom asked for by the patient/service user, nearly always by the judgment of the professional.

Our next finding was that the individuals for which CIP was used had many and varied social and health problems, most often involving some form of substance abuse in combination with some kind of mental health problem, and often one or several of a range of physical health problems. Most had several kinds of social problems involving personal economy, employment or other regular activities (only one had any form of employment), housing, criminality, prostitution, or family relations [23].

Representation at CIP meetings was fairly even among social service assessment and healthcare's addiction treatment and outpatient psychiatric care, but social service care provision and primary health care were represented less often. There were many CIPs in which the professionals at the meeting did not have a mandate to make the formal decisions which were discussed, and user participation was seldom documented (other than that the patient/service user had been present at the meeting).

An additional significant finding was that the CIPs were seldom specifically motivated and most often merely listed the person's needs and which care and interventions were ongoing or planned. Discussions of the individual's needs and which care/interventions were suggested and agreed upon appeared to have been rudimentary [23].

Findings in the second file study were similar in all significant respects, despite the different selection of files [25]. Our analysis was that the individuals for whom CIP was used did have complex problems, as was the intention with CIP, but that CIP was used unsystematically. This led us to characterize CIP as an unsystematic form of interagency meeting, placing it in the lower half of Andersson et al.'s scale [32]. There was some evidence of supporting structures for CIP in the organizations, particularly in the second study, but it was questionable whether the supporting structures were adequate to achieve a high degree of collaboration. Instead, considering the uneven representation and professional discretion and the unclear level of user participation, we analyzed the degree of collaboration as low to moderate, using our modified version of Axelsson and Bihari Axelsson's conceptual framework (**Figure 1**).

3.2 The interview study: Secondary characters, patient vulnerability, and organizational uncertainty

Twenty qualitative interviews were conducted in seven local authorities with professionals who had experience of CIP. Fifteen interviewees were with professionals in the social service and five from their collaborative partners in psychiatric mental health care. The findings from the file studies were used as a basis for the interview guide. The interviews were transcribed and coded into domains, categories, sub-categories, and themes [26, 27]. Qualitative content analysis was used in this process, in which the two authors continually consulted each other with the intention of interpreting both the manifest content and the latent content in the interview material [33].

A first analysis focused on how the professionals see user involvement/user participation in CIP [23]. Our starting point was Laitila et al.'s definition of user involvement, which is that users/patients are respected and listened to and can influence their own care in cooperation with professionals [34]. In a systematic review of research on shared decision-making, Francis, Johnson, and Wilson concluded that clinicians need to be able to trust that their organization supports and prioritizes user involvement, and that service users want to be involved and make requests [35]. We based our theoretical analysis on Lipsky's concept of "street-level bureaucracy," first published in 1980, according to which front-line workers such as social workers and healthcare professionals use their professional discretion to act as advocates for individual service users/patients, while at the same time controlling users/patients so that they do not make demands which cannot be met within available resources [36].

We then expanded the analysis to include the professionals' broader experience of CIP [27]. According to the governmental proposition, the aim of CIP is to improve collaboration among organizations [22]. We used the theory of institutional isomorphism, as conceptualized by DiMaggio and Powell, to understand how change has or has not been achieved through CIP. DiMaggio and Powell describe *coercive, mimetic*, and *normative* mechanisms of isomorphism [37, 38]. CIP as an instrument of collaboration can be described as a form of coercive isomorphism driven by legislation and accompanying regulations [39]. Mimetic isomorphism refers to imitation of what is regarded as successive models from other organizations. Mimetic activities can be recognized under the terms of benchmarking and networking activities. Normative isomorphism occurs when change is dependent on professionalization. Whether or not organizational change occurs depends on the balance between these mechanisms of isomorphism [37].

As mentioned above, findings from the interview study have been previously published in two articles [26, 27]. A simplified representation of the findings is shown in **Table 1**.

Concerning user involvement, we found two principal themes [26, 27]. The first was "The user/patient as principal subject or as secondary character." The categories and sub-categories concerned whether the focus of the meeting was on the user/patient's needs, or was the user/patient (as one interviewee expressed it) a kind of "secondary character"; whether the user/patient was an active participant or was not included in the discussions; and, as a third aspect, whether family members (in those meetings when they were present) were a support for the user, or whether the family members took so much space that the meeting became more for their sake than for the individual's.

The second theme was "The user/patient as vulnerable among experts." The first category concerned the user's role, where the professionals tended to push responsibility for the user's needs over to the other organizations present ("the user as a problem for someone else"), or, as in some cases, tried to educate the user to have more realistic expectations for help ("the user as the object of a pedagogical effort"). The other category concerned the user's satisfaction or frustration with the help he/she received.

Interview domains	Themes	
The user/patient's participation in CIP meetings The user/patient's position in collaboration	The user as a prime subject or a secondary character	The user as vulnerable among experts
The purpose of SIP The execution of CIP	CIP in action—the model in practice	Organizational uncertainty

Table 1.
Simplified table representing findings from the interview study. More complete tables are included in Matscheck and Piuva [26] and Matscheck and Piuva [27].

The broader analysis also found two principal themes [27]. The first was "CIP in action—the model in practice." Here, the focus was either on CIP for the sake of the user/patient, or on CIP as a mandatory tool. If CIP was for the sake of the user/patient, the focus was on seeing to it that he/she got answers to his/her questions and on clarification of "who does what." If focus was on the mandatory nature of CIP, then the different organizations were "forced" to meet and discuss what was or was not working, in which case the issue was whether CIP does, in fact, solve problems in collaboration.

The other theme was "Organizational uncertainty." CIP requires a lot of administration and documentation, and there was often a lack of efficient routines. CIP was meant to solve conflicts but was often hindered by the tendency for all parts to see only their own perspective, rather than the individual's entire situation. On the organizational level, local collaboration agreements established collaboration boards, but there was little to indicate that the collaboration boards took a significant role in supporting CIP. In some local authorities, local models had been developed to try to improve collaboration for the target group. But in one local authority, a model which had been seen as working well had been discontinued when CIP was legislated, which appears to have to worsened rather than improved collaboration.

3.3 Other research on CIP: Service user participation and shared decision-making

The research on CIP which has started later than the authors' project has primarily focused on service user participation and has come to similar results. Nordström and colleagues [29] studied the use of CIP with people with intellectual disabilities and found a gap between policy and practice where service user participation is considered by professionals to be an important goal, but difficult to put into practice. Jones, Knutsson and Schön [28] also studied service user participation in CIP, focusing on shared decision-making (SDM) as a possible way forward, but found the same kinds of difficulties as we have found in our research.

4. Discussion

The legislation which created CIP was based on an analysis which showed that previous attempts to stimulate collaboration around individuals with concomitant mental health problems and substance abuse had, as with other groups, not been adequate to achieve necessary change. CIP is an attempt to scale up collaboration and reach a wider group of patients/service users by coercive means, that is, by making CIP mandatory "when needed."

Our findings indicate that CIP has been used unevenly, but also that, in those cases where CIP has been used, it has in fact been used for individuals for whom collaboration is necessary. The individuals in the case files we have studied had need of help from social care and psychiatric mental health and/or substance abuse care, and also from somatic health care as well as, in some cases, other societal organizations. Responsibility for and provision of these kinds of care was fragmented, divided among several sectors and organizations and a variety of professions.

Nevertheless, analysis of our findings indicates only a low to moderate degree of collaboration, which we have shown in our modified version of Axelsson and Bihari Axelssons' conceptual scheme [23] (**Figure 1**). Information concerning the individual was provided, but deeper discussions of the individual's needs and possible long-term interventions or treatment were unusual.

The need for collaboration can be addressed by developing structures for organizational support. In an earlier research project, Matscheck and Axelsson showed an example of how Axelsson and Bihari Axelsson's conceptual scheme can be appropriate to analyze how contacts can be established at different organizational levels, between organizations and across sectors [40]. In the case of CIP, local collaboration agreements had been reached in all the local authorities we studied, which is in accordance with legislative requirements. Nevertheless, our findings show few indications that these local agreements have been used as a means of providing organizational support for CIP. Instead, interview findings indicate that the professionals most often have been left on their own with the problems involved in collaboration on the level of treatment and provision, which they are expected to solve in the presence of the user/patient.

CIP has also been presented as a means of increasing patients' and service users' involvement in their own care. But although the individual was present at almost all CIP meetings, and despite interviewees' assertions that CIPs are done "for the sake of the user," indications of actual influence over care were limited.

In sum, the ambition of scaling up collaboration appears only to have been achieved to a limited degree. Professionals have been left with inadequate organizational support, leaving tendencies to competition between agencies to dominate the reality of CIP in practice. The additional ambition to combine increased collaboration with user/patient involvement has also been difficult to realize.

CIP was introduced as an attempt to change the organizational situation which had led to lack of collaboration between different welfare sectors, in this case between psychiatric mental health care and care and treatment of alcohol and drug addiction. Following the logics of neo-institutionalism, organizational change is powered by the balance between legislation (coercive isomorphism), mimicry of successful practitioners (mimetic isomorphism), and professional knowledge (normative isomorphism). The fact that CIP is coercive can be perceived as degrading by professions who usually operate in environments with high normative isomorphism, especially in medical disciplines where research results govern activities, which may have led to passive resistance to using the model.

Within the social work sector in Sweden, results of research have had limited influence on organizational changes and working methods. In the social welfare sectors, the economic policy paradigm of New Public Management continues to dominate. In the organizations which we have examined there were examples of mimetic isomorphism before the legislation on CIP, such as networking, local development projects, and joint professional conferences. The limited use of professional and local development projects can be understood as a legislative hampering of mimetic isomorphism.

Difficulties in collaboration appear to be especially pronounced in Sweden. In connection with mental health, it has been difficult in practice to draw clear lines between the different organization's responsibilities, both within the healthcare sector between psychiatric care and primary care, and among the social services, the state's social insurance, and the state employment service. The purchaser-provider split, with private care contracted on the provider side, sometimes with the use in-hired doctors, has added to the difficulties [12]. But the problem of fragmentation of care is nevertheless known to be international [4, 24, 32], so the difficulties encountered with CIP can hardly be said to be unique.

The difficulty in increasing service user/patient participation is also not surprising. In a newly published observational study from the Netherlands, for example, researchers analyzed user participation in recorded meetings with professionals from multiple organizations [41]. They found that it proved difficult to make the individual's voice central, and that divisions between the individual and the several professions often arose. These kinds of findings confirm the difficulty in realizing ambitions for increased participation which we found in studying CIP. In our analysis, we found that, in the environment of the CIP meeting, the street-level bureaucrat's gatekeeper role in relation to the patient/service user easily takes precedence over the role of advocate for the individual, leaving the service user/patient as what one interviewee called a "secondary character."

It appears that something more is needed. In an earlier paper concerning collaboration around children and young people, the first author and a colleague introduced the idea of "collaboration competence" [42]. Similarly formulated ideas have occasionally turned up in academic papers [43], but on the whole, there appears not to exist a general concept that expresses the idea that to collaborate well, professionals at all levels need to possess a particular kind of competence.

What the authors are naming "collaboration competence" has to do with developing the ability to handle to the processes involved in collaboration. Developing collaboration competence in welfare organizations would involve such issues as learning more about how collaborative partners work in their professions and about the legal and organizational conditions which steer what they can offer the patient/service user. It would also involve common training sessions to handle the discussions which arise in collaborative meetings, such as in CIP meetings or in other forms of collaboration. It could also involve regular "arenas" for communication and discussions among collaborative partners [40]. In order to successfully develop such collaboration competence, it would also need to be an important element in educational programs for professionals in health care, social work, and other welfare sectors.

This kind of training has been attempted in the regional and local authorities which we studied, but only in 1- or 2-day sessions and in most cases only in connection with the initial implementation of the CIP model [25]. It is not a prioritized subject in health care or social work education in Sweden. We suggest that much more attention is needed to the issues of collaboration competence and supporting structures if a model such as CIP is to have greater impact in achieving change in the direction of integrated care.

5. Conclusions

In a development similar to that in other countries, there has been limited impact in Sweden for models for collaboration such as case management and team-based models such as ACT and FACT. This has led to an attempt to scale up collaboration by legislating mandatory use of a more general model, the coordinated individual plan (CIP). The authors' research indicates that implementation of CIP has also had limited impact, leading to low-to-moderate levels of collaboration over sectors, organizations, and professions. An additional ambition with CIP was to increase patients' and service users' involvement in their own care, but findings indicate limited impact also in this area. Other existing research on CIP has led to similar findings.

The authors conclude that, if models for scaling up collaboration such as CIP are to have greater impact, organizational structures to support the model need to be developed and utilized to a greater degree. Directors, managers, and workers in relevant departments and clinics need to be engaged in furthering collaboration across sectors, organizations, and professions. If in turn such engagement is to be achieved, the authors propose the concept "collaboration competence," by which is meant the use of education and training to develop necessary skills to handle the processes necessary for collaboration. We suggest that the development of this kind of competence would encourage normative and mimetic isomorphism, rather than coercive isomorphism, within professional organizations, enabling greater impact for collaborative models.

Acknowledgements

The authors would like to thank FoU Nordost (RD Northeast Stockholm) and FoU Nordväst (RD Northwest Stockholm), especially Lisbeth Eriksson and Martin Åberg, for their contributions to portions of this project.

The project was completed without external funding.

Conflict of interest

The authors declare no conflict of interest.

Author details

David Robert Matscheck* and Katarina Piuva
Department of Social Work, Stockholm University, Stockholm, Sweden

*Address all correspondence to: david.matscheck@gmail.com

References

[1] Börjeson B. Förstå Socialt Arbete [Understand Social Work]. Malmö: Liber; 2011. p. 39. 560 p

[2] SFS 1982:763 Hälso- och Sjukvårdslagen [Swedish Code of States 1982:763. Health and Medical Care Services Act]. Amended SFS 2009:979, SFS 2013:302

[3] SFS 2001:453. Socialtjänstlagen [Swedish Code of States 2001:453. Social Service Act.] Amended SFS 2003:407, SFS 2003:412, SFS 2009:981, SFS 2013:303

[4] Miller C, Ahmad Y. Collaboration and partnership: An effective response to complexity and fragmentation or a solution built on sand? International Journal of Sociology and Social Policy. 2000;**20**:1-38. DOI: 10.1108/01443330010789151

[5] Klingemann J, Welbel M, Priebe S, Giacco D, Matanov A, Lorant V, et al. Personal continuity versus specialization of care approaches in mental healthcare: Experiences of patients and clinicians—Results of the qualitative study in five European countries. Social Psychiatry and Psychiatric Epidemiology. 2020;**55**:205-216. DOI: 10.1007/s00127-019-01757-z

[6] Raeymaeckers P. A specialist's perspective on the value of generalist practice: A qualitative network analysis. Journal of Social Work. 2016;**16**(5):610-626. DOI: 10.1177/1468017316644693

[7] Pollitt C, Bouckaert G. Public Management Reform—A Comparative Analysis: New Public Management Governance, and the Neo-Weberian State. 3rd ed. Oxford: Oxford University Press; 2011. 367 p

[8] Hood C. A public management for all seasons. Public Administration. 1991;**69**:3-19

[9] Shanks E, Lundström T, Wiklund S. Middle managers in social work. Professional identity and management in a marketized welfare state. British Journal of Social Work. 2015;**45**:443-460. DOI: 10.1093/bjsw/bcu061

[10] Sallnäs M. Introduktion—Socialtjänstmarknaden under radarn [Introduction—The social service market under the radar]. In: Sallnäs M, Wiklund S, editors. Socialtjänstmarknaden—Om marknadsorientering och konkurrensutsättning av individ- och familjeomsorgen [The Social Service Market—On market orientation and competition in personal social services]. Stockholm: Liber; 2018. pp. 14-29

[11] Horsfall J, Cleary M, Hunt GE, Walter G. Psychosocial treatments for people with co-occurring severe mental illness and substance use disorders (double diagnosis): A review of empirical evidence. Harvard Review of Psychiatry. 2009;**17**(1):24-34. DOI: 10.1080/10673220902724599

[12] Piuva K. Happy without reason—Mental illness and the 'right' to happiness in Sweden. In: Marklund C, editor. All Well in the Welfare State? Welfare, Well-Being and the Politics of Happiness, NordWel Studies in Historical Welfare State Research. Vol. 5. Helsinki: University of Helsinki; 2013. pp. 55-81

[13] Lindqvist R, Rosenberg D, Fredén L. Den svenska psykiatrireformen i nordisk belysning [The Swedish mental health reform in the Nordic context]. Socialmedicinsk Tidskrift [Journal of Social Medicine]. 2011;**88**(6):524-533

[14] Arvidsson H. The development of needs in a Group of Severely Mentally ill—A 10 year follow-up study after the 1995 Swedish mental health care reform. Social Psychiatry and Psychiatric Epidemiology. 2008;**43**(9):705-713. DOI: 10.1007/s00127-008-0356-7

[15] Markström U, Lindqvist R. Establishment of community mental health systems in a postdeinstitutional era: A study of organizational structures and service provision in Sweden. Journal of Social Work in Disability & Rehabilitation. 2015;**14**(2):124-144. DOI: 10.1080/1536710X.2015.1014535

[16] Oscarsson L. Missbrukarvården och samhället [Care of substance abuse and society]. In: Official Government Report SOU 2011:6, Missbruket, Kunskapen, Vården [Substance Abuse, Scientific Knowledge, Care], Missbruksutredningens Forskningsbilaga [Research Supplement to the Official Government Report on Substance Abuse]. Stockholm: Statens Offentliga Utredningar; 2011

[17] Bergmark M, Bejerholm U, Svensson B, Markström U. Complex interventions and interorganisational relationships: Examining core implementation components of assertive community treatment. International Journal of Integrated Care. 2018;**18**(4):11, 1-11. DOI: 10.5334ijic.3547

[18] Bjerkan J, Richter M, Grimsmo A, Hellesø R, Brender J. Integrated care in Norway: The state of affairs years after regulation by law. International Journal of Integrated Care. 2011;**2011**:11. DOI: 10.5334/ijic.530

[19] Simpson A, Hannigan B, Coffey M, Barlow S, Cohen R, Jones A, et al. Recovery-focused care planning and coordination in England and Wales: A cross-national mixed methods comparative case study. BMC Psychiatry. 2016;**16**:147. DOI: 10.1186/s12888-016-0858-x

[20] NHS (National Health Service). Care Programme Approach. Official NHS England Position Statement. 2022. Available from: https://www.england.nhs.uk/wp-content/uploads/2021/07/B0526-care-programme-approach-position-statement-v2.pdf [Accessed: January 9, 2025]

[21] SFS 2009:981. Amendment to Socialtjänstlagen SFS 2001:453 [Swedish Code of States 2001:453. Social Service Act.]

[22] Governmental Proposition 2008/09:193. Regeringens Proposition—Vissa Psykiatrifrågor m.m. [The Swedish Government's Proposition—Certain Questions Concerning Psychiatry etc.]

[23] Matscheck D, Piuva K, Eriksson L, Åberg M. The coordinated individual plan—Is this a solution for complex organizations to handle complex needs? Nordic Social Work Research. 2019;**9**(1):55-71. DOI: 10.1080/2156857X.2018.1489886© 2018

[24] Bihari AR, Axelsson S. Integration and collaboration in public health—A conceptual framework. The International Journal of Health Planning and Management. 2006;**21**(1):75-88. Available from: https://doi-org.ezp.sub.su.se/10.1002/hpm.826

[25] Matscheck D, Piuva K. Integrated care for individuals with mental illness and substance abuse—The example of the coordinated individual plan in Sweden. European Journal of Social Work. 2022;**25**(2):341-354. DOI: 10.1080/13691457.2020.1843409

[26] Matscheck D, Piuva K. In the Center or Caught in the Middle?—Social

workers' and health care professionals' views on user involvement in Coordinated Individual Plans in Sweden. Health & Social Care in the Community. 2022;**30**:1077-1085. DOI: 10.1111/hsc.13311

[27] Matscheck D, Piuva K. Exploring the effectiveness of the coordinated individual plan in Sweden: Challenges and opportunities for collaborative care. Nordic Social Work Research. 2023. Available from: https://doi-org.ezp.sub.su.se/10.1080/2156857X.2023.2281977

[28] Jones A, Knutsson O, Schön U-K. Coordinated individual care planning and shared decision-making: Staff perspectives within the comorbidity field of practice. European Journal of Social Work. 2022;**25**(2):355-367. DOI: 10.1080/13691457.2021.201664

[29] Nordström L, Lassinantti K, Carlsson OU, Almqvist A-L. Service-user participation in coordinated planning, from the perspective of involved professionals. Disability & Society. 2024;**39**(12):3212-3234. DOI: 10.1080/09687599.2023.2255736

[30] Nordström E, Josephson I, Hedberg B, Kjellström S. Agenda för samverkan eller verksamhetens agenda?—Om professionellas erfarenheter av samverkan enligt samordnad individuell plan [Agenda for collaboration or collaboration parties' agenda?—On professionals' experiences of collaboration according to the coordinated individual plan]. Socialvetenskaplig Tidskrift. 2016;**23**(1):37-57. DOI: 10.3384/SVT.2016.23.1.2334

[31] Lawrence PA, Lorsch JW. Organization and Environment: Managing Differentiation and Integration. Boston, MA: Harvard University Press; 1967. 279 p

[32] Andersson J, Ahgren B, Bihari AS, Eriksson A, Axelsson R. Organizational approaches to collaboration in vocational rehabilitation—An international literature review. International Journal of Integrated Care. 2011;**11**:1-10. DOI: 10.5334/ijic.670

[33] Elo S, Kyngäs H. The qualitative content analysis process. Journal of Advanced Nursing. 2008;**62**(1):107-115. DOI: 10.1111/j.1365-2648.2007.04569.x

[34] Laitila M, Nummelin J, Kortteisto T, Pitkänen A. Service users' views regarding user involvement in mental health services: A qualitative study. Archives of Psychiatric Nursing. 2018;**32**(5):695-701. DOI: 10.1016/j.apnu.2018.03.009

[35] Francis CJ, Johnson A, Wilson RL. Supported decision-making interventions in mental healthcare: A systematic review of current evidence and implementation barriers. Health Expectations. 2024;**27**:e14001. DOI: 10.1111/hex.14001

[36] Lipsky M. Street-Level Bureaucracy—Dilemmas of the Individual in Public Services. Updated ed. New York: Russell Sage Foundation; 2010. 275 p

[37] DiMaggio JP, Powell WW. The iron cage revisited: Institutional isomorphism and collective rationality in organizational fields. American Sociological Review. 1983;**48**(2):147-160. DOI: 10.2307/2095101

[38] DiMaggio JP, Powell WW. Introduction. In: Powell WW, DiMaggio P, editors. The New Institutionalism in Organizational Analysis. Chicago: The University of Chicago Press; 1991. 275 p

[39] Bergmark Å, Germundsson N, Lundström T, Stranz H. Ringar på vattnet—Om socialtjänstens individ- och

familjeomsorg i samverkan. [Ripples on the water—Collaboration and personal social services]. Socionomens Forskningssupplement. 2017;**28**(1):31-38. ISSN 0283-1929

[40] Matscheck D, Axelsson R. Arenas for contact. Scandinavian Journal of Public Administration. 2012;**16**(2):93-113. DOI: 10.58235/sjpa.v16i2.16228

[41] Nouwen C, Van Hattum M, Driesen I. Multiple alliances and client participation during joint client meetings: An observational study. European Social Work Research. 2024;**2**:294-311. DOI: 10.1332/27551768Y2024D000000020

[42] Fleetwood C, Matscheck D. BUS-avtalet—En fråga om samverkans-kompetens [The children with special needs agreement—A question of collaboration competence]. In: Bihari AR, Axelsson S, editors. Folkhälsa I Samverkan [Public Health in Collaboration]. Lund: Studentlitteratur; 2007. pp. 163-181

[43] Getha-Taylor H. Identifying collaborative competencies. Review of Public Personnel Administration. 2008;**28**(2):103-119. DOI: 10.1177/0734371X08315434

Chapter 3

Art Therapy Applications in Hemodialysis Patients: A Bibliometric Analysis Study

Songül Mollaoğlu and Mukadder Mollaoğlu

Abstract

This study is a Bibliometrix analysis conducted in the field of health between 2014 and 2025 using the keywords "hemodialysis," "art therapy," and "chronic kidney failure." A search was conducted in the Scopus database to access relevant articles. The keywords "hemodialysis," "art therapy," and "chronic kidney failure" were used in the search. As a result, a total of 29,242 studies were identified, and 402 studies meeting the criteria were included for analysis. The research was analyzed and visualized using Biblioshiny, the web interface provider of the R-based Bibliometrix analysis program. The number of studies on the use of art therapy in hemodialysis patients peaked in 2024. The United States produced the highest number of publications. In conceptual networks, the theme "Chronic Kidney Failure" stood out. In the document co-citation network, the paper published by Cupisti was prominent, Fouque was the most productive author, and the journal with the most publications was the *Journal of Renal Nutrition*. Mayo Clinic was the university with the highest number of publications. The review of studies conducted in the last 11 years on hemodialysis and art therapy showed that effective interventions for improving and enhancing health have been tested. Additionally, while art therapy emerges as a supportive treatment method for alleviating symptoms in chronic kidney failure, the academic output in this field is still insufficient. In conclusion, this bibliometric analysis provides valuable information for researchers in terms of strategic planning, developing collaborations, and identifying gaps in the literature.

Keywords: hemodialysis, art therapy, chronic kidney failure, bibliometrix analysis, scopus, biblioshiny

1. Introduction

Chronic kidney disease (CKD) is a rapidly growing global public health problem in the twenty-first century. According to Global Burden of Disease Study data, CKD directly contributed to 1.2 million deaths and is expected to become one of the top five causes of death by 2040 [1].

For patients who develop end-stage renal disease (ESRD), the most common renal replacement therapy is hemodialysis. Hemodialysis sessions—performed at least two to three times per week for 3–5 hours each—profoundly change patients' lives not only through biomedical but also social, psychological, and economic impacts. Numerous studies have shown that dialysis patients have higher rates of depression, anxiety, adjustment disorders, and even trauma-like symptoms than the general population [2, 3]. Meta-analytic findings indicate that the prevalence of depression among hemodialysis patients ranges from 22 to 39%. Depression and anxiety adversely affect not only subjective quality of life but also mortality, hospitalization rates, and treatment adherence [4, 5]. Today, evaluating patients only through biological parameters is considered inadequate in nephrology practice, and a patient-centered care approach has gained importance. Integrative treatment methods such as art therapy, which support medical treatment in patient management, have also become important.

Art therapy is a psychotherapy approach that helps individuals express their inner experiences, develop awareness, and gain psychological flexibility through creative processes [6]. Different art forms such as painting, sculpture, collage, writing, drama, and music allow exploration of emotions at a symbolic level, going beyond the limits of verbal expression. Art therapy is applied with goals such as strengthening emotion regulation skills, developing coping strategies, supporting identity and self-esteem, and facilitating meaning-making processes, especially in individuals with chronic illnesses [4, 6]. Although research on art therapy among hemodialysis patients is relatively limited, interest has been increasing. Early studies in the 2000s began with case reports and qualitative explorations, while the post-2010 period has seen the addition of quasi-experimental and randomized controlled designs.

In recent years, research on art therapy for hemodialysis patients has been steadily increasing. Studies in Spain demonstrate the increasing diversity of art therapy within the healthcare field. Analyses in social work highlight that art therapy research has expanded beyond the Western world and is being applied to hemodialysis patients in countries such as South Korea, Italy, and Chile. Global bibliometric studies on hemodialysis reveal increasing academic interest in art therapy for this patient group. Art therapy is being implemented for hemodialysis patients in an increasing number of countries and is receiving increasing attention in the academic literature [7–9].

Art therapy stands out as an important element of holistic care models due to its feasibility and potential effects in hemodialysis patients. However, the existing literature faces issues such as methodological diversity, sample limitations, and a lack of cultural context. Over the past 20 years, there has been growing research on the effects of art therapy in other chronic disease groups such as oncology, dementia, chronic pain, and diabetes. Systematic reviews and meta-analyses have shown that art therapy provides benefits such as reducing anxiety and depression symptoms, improving quality of life, and supporting treatment adherence [10, 11].

In this study, there was a need to evaluate art therapy practices in hemodialysis patients with chronic kidney disease through systematic analyses and a bibliometric perspective to shed light on research gaps.

1.1 Significance and aim of the study

This study is thought to have the potential to help academics understand current and future research trends by revealing conceptual richness, thereby enabling more innovative and creative research. In this context, the aim of the study is to conduct a bibliometric analysis of articles published on the effects of art therapy in patients undergoing hemodialysis using the R-based Bibliometrix program.

1.2 Research questions

- **Q1:** What is the growth trend and citation status of articles on the effects of art therapy in hemodialysis patients?
- **Q2:** Who are the leading authors with the highest citations in the field?
- **Q3:** Which journals, documents, countries, and institutions have the most citations?
- **Q4:** What are the key research points and thematic investigations in this field?
- **Q5:** Which publication has the highest number of citations?

1.3 Contributions of the study

In this study, bibliometric analyses for articles on the effects of art therapy in hemodialysis patients were created using quantitative tools such as Bibliometrix, Biblioshiny (a web-based interface for R), and VOSviewer 1.6.20. The study provided a conceptual framework for publications on the effects of art therapy in hemodialysis patients and identified the most influential articles and productive contributors in the field.

The findings of the study may help researchers better understand current and future research trends on the effects of art therapy in hemodialysis patients.

2. Literature review

Table 1 includes studies examining the prevalence and impact of hemodialysis and art therapy in practice. **Table 1** summarizes bibliometric analyses of research in the field of hemodialysis or art therapy.

3. Method

In this study, the bibliometric analysis method was applied. First introduced by Pritchard, bibliometric analysis is defined as "the quantitative and qualitative analysis of published academic literature to track the development of a specific research field over time." In other words, bibliometric analysis aims to profile the body of work within a scientific field or discipline, systematically demonstrating the development of scientific knowledge [12].

Bibliometric analysis is a powerful technique for tracking research trends and discoveries. Its process steps are as follows:

Step 1: Selecting a database.

Scopus and Google Scholar are among the accessible data sources.

Step 2: Filtering information in the database.

Information is retrieved from the chosen database and evaluated by filtering with "inclusion" and "exclusion" criteria.

Step 3: Choosing software for bibliometric analysis.

One or more software tools such as RStudio (Biblioshiny) and VOSviewer 1.6.20 are selected to conduct the bibliometric analysis.

Authors	Year	Key words	Time range	Number of publications reviewed	Database	Softwares used
Liu et al.	2021	Art therapy; Bibliometric analysis; Co-occurrence analysis; Health and well-being; Therapeutic method; Children; adolescent; elderly; Psychotherapy; Virtual reality	1946–2021	799	Scopus	VOSviewer and Biblioshiny
Natalia Rodriguez Novo et al.	2021	Art therapy, Bibliometric, Trend analysis, Visual arts, Health	1994–2020	563	WoS	Biblioshiny
Jia-Fen Wu and Chi-Yang Chung	2023	Art therapy, Bibliometric analysis, Children, Historiography, Intervention	1990–2020	87	WoS	Biblioshiny, Social Sciences Citation Index (SSCI)
Carmen Lopez-Escribano et al.	2023	Art therapy Visual art Intervention Assessment Bibliometric analysis Spanish	2011–2021	160	Scopus, Web of Science ve Google Scholar	Biblioshiny
Yufen Wang ve ark	2024	Bibliometric, CiteSpace software, Hemodialysis, VOSviewer	2002–2023	1019	WoS	VOSviewer, ve Biblioshiny
Zi-Ran Sun et al.	2023	Hemodialysis; quality of life; Web of Science; bibliometric analysis introduction	1985–2022	1597	WoS	Biblioshiny
Yoo Jin Lee et al.	2021	Analysis, Hemodialysis, Publications	1969–2019	100	WoS	Biblioshiny
Lily Kresnowati et al.	2024	Diabetic kidney disease, Bibliometric, Hemodialysis, Health insurance, Machine learning	2010–2022	2199	Scopus	VOSviewer, ve Biblioshiny

Table 1.
Bibliometric analyses related to hemodialysis or art therapy.

Step 4: Defining the bibliometric analysis.

Through performance analysis of the studies, the following elements are identified: main information, annual publication trends, annual citation trends, three-field plots, journal status, membership status, author profiles, country-level analyses, and article characteristics.

Scientific mapping visually reveals relationships among texts, similarities or differences between topics, publication trends, and the significance of key concepts [13]. For this purpose, conceptual structure maps, thematic maps, trending topics, and keyword co-occurrence analyses are applied. The process steps of bibliometric analysis are summarized in **Figure 1**.

In **Figure 1**, the first step shows that the international *Scopus* database was used as the data source for this study. Scopus is considered the most powerful search engine in the field of social sciences. Although it is fundamentally similar to other databases, Scopus is regarded as a comprehensive index of the existing social science literature. It is widely used by many authors for comparable studies [14–16]. The Scopus database includes journal titles, h-index matrices, citation matrices, and other features that enable effective bibliometric analyses, and it is equipped with operational functions [17].

For the second step, the query period was set as 2014–2025 (January), and the data were downloaded on June 15, 2025 (**Table 2**).

The data were downloaded in .csv format and sorted from the most cited to the least cited.

The flowchart of the first and second steps of the data collection process is shown in **Figure 2**. The identification, screening, and inclusion criteria represent the data search steps followed in **Figure 2**. In the final stage, 402 studies were included for review.

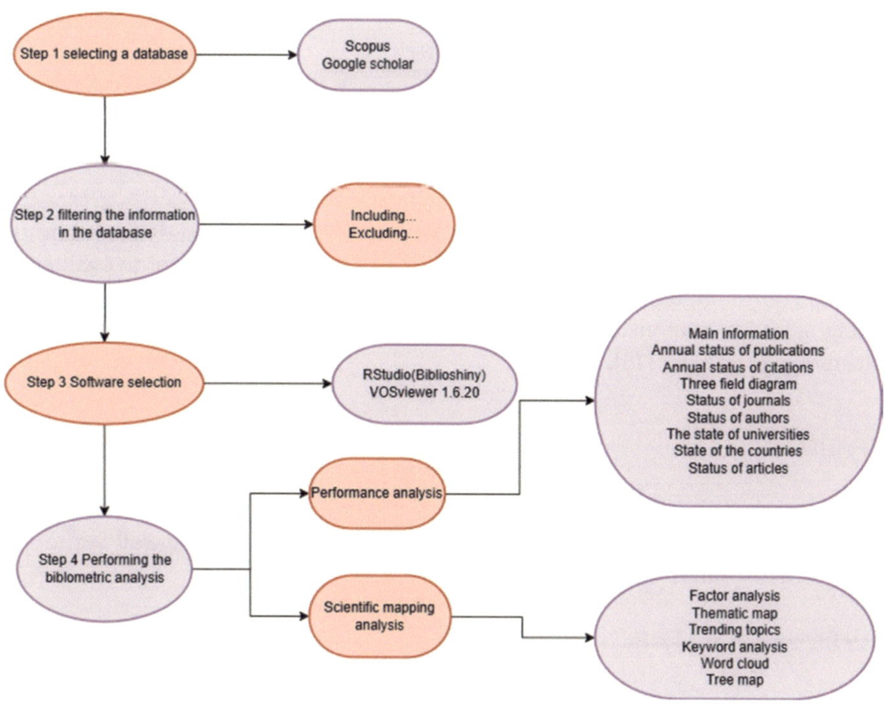

Figure 1.
Flowchart of the bibliometric analysis process.

Included	Excluded
Keywords: "hemodialysis", "art therapy", and "chronic kidney failure"	Reviews and conference proceedings published on preprint websites, book chapters, articles or reviews, as well as comments, editorials, and letters
Document type: Article Publication language: English Publication format: Journal Publication year: 2014–2025	

Table 2.
Filtering information in the scopus database.

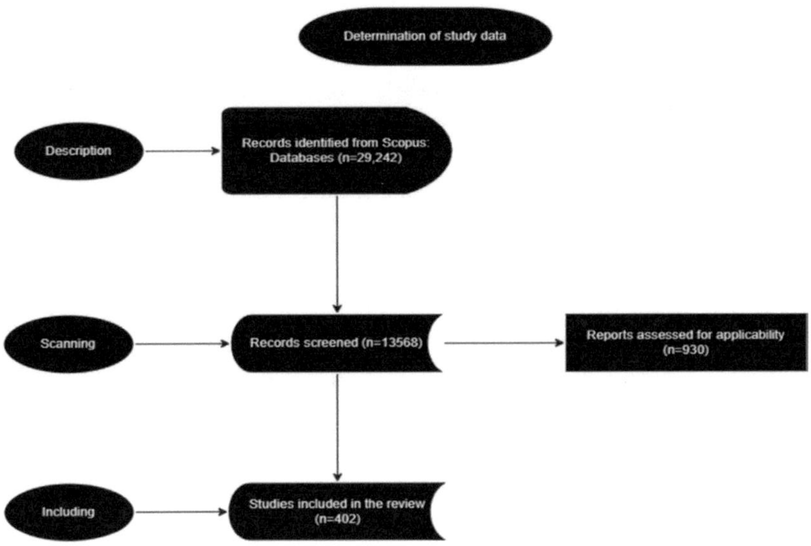

Figure 2.
The flowchart of the first and second steps of the data collection process is shown in **Figure 2**.

As the third step, the *R Bibliometrix* package was used in this study for bibliometric analysis [18]. In the final step, performance analysis was employed to evaluate the publications through detailed descriptive analysis and scientific mapping analysis, enabling researchers to visually explore and analyze the data and communicate their results more effectively [13].

4. Results

Below are the bibliometric analysis results of studies conducted using the keywords "hemodialysis," "art therapy," and "chronic kidney failure," as well as the analyses and examinations related to the process.

4.1 Performance analysis

A detailed descriptive analysis of the publications was performed, including an assessment of the annual publication growth rate and an estimate of the average number of citations per publication. A diagram known as a *Sankey diagram* was used to compare three different fields: identifying which journal had the most publications and citations, as well as determining the institutions and documents with the highest publication and citation counts.

The study also identified and analyzed the author and country with the largest output in terms of publications, citations, and data performance analysis [13].

4.1.1 General overview of the database

Biblioshiny was used to perform descriptive analyses of the impact of chemotherapy on quality of life. **Figure 3** presents the general information in the database. From the 29,242 articles in the Scopus database published between 2014 and 2025, 402 articles meeting the criteria were included for evaluation.

Between 2014 and 2025, 402 articles on the impact of art therapy in hemodialysis patients, published in 118 sources (journals) indexed in the Scopus database, were evaluated. Publications increased at an annual rate of 2.49%, with an average age of 5.03 years and an average of 13.9 citations per article. Among 2286 authors, 11 published as single authors. The rate of international co-authorship in the documents accounted for 19.15% of the total.

4.1.2 Annual publication growth

Figure 4 shows the evolution over time of the documents included in the bibliometric analysis conducted using the keywords "hemodialysis," "art therapy," and "chronic kidney failure."

In the distribution by year of studies conducted using the keywords "hemodialysis," "art therapy," and "chronic kidney failure," there were 28 studies in 2023, 63 in 2024, and 38 in 2025. The highest number of publications occurred in 2024.

4.1.3 Annual average citations

Figure 5 shows the annual citation trends in the bibliometric analysis of studies using the keywords "hemodialysis," "art therapy," and "chronic kidney failure."

Figure 5 illustrates the changes in the number of citations over time. The total citations per article were 0.61 in 2025, 1.68 in 2024, and 4.54 in 2023.

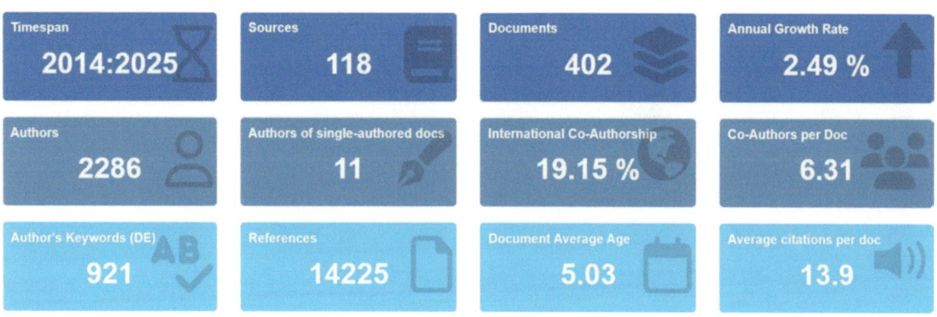
Timespan
2014:2025
Sources
118
Documents
402
Annual Growth Rate
2.49 %
Authors
2286
Authors of single-authored docs
11
International Co-Authorship
19.15 %
Co-Authors per Doc
6.31
Author's Keywords (DE)
921
References
14225
Document Average Age
5.03
Average citations per doc
13.9

Figure 3.
Main information.

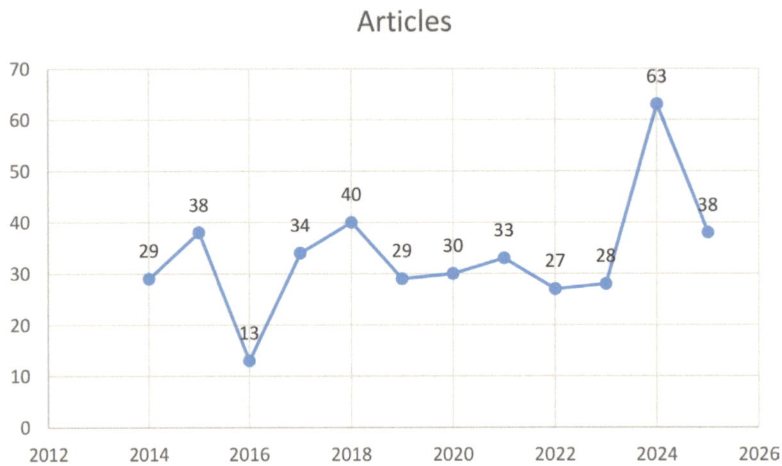

Figure 4.
Annual distribution of publications.

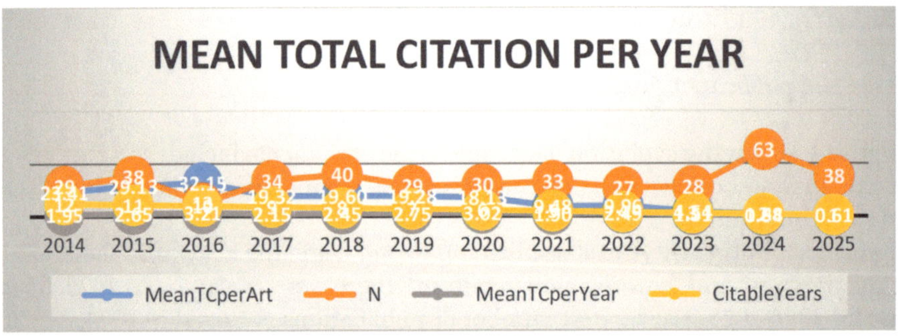

Figure 5.
Annual citation trends.

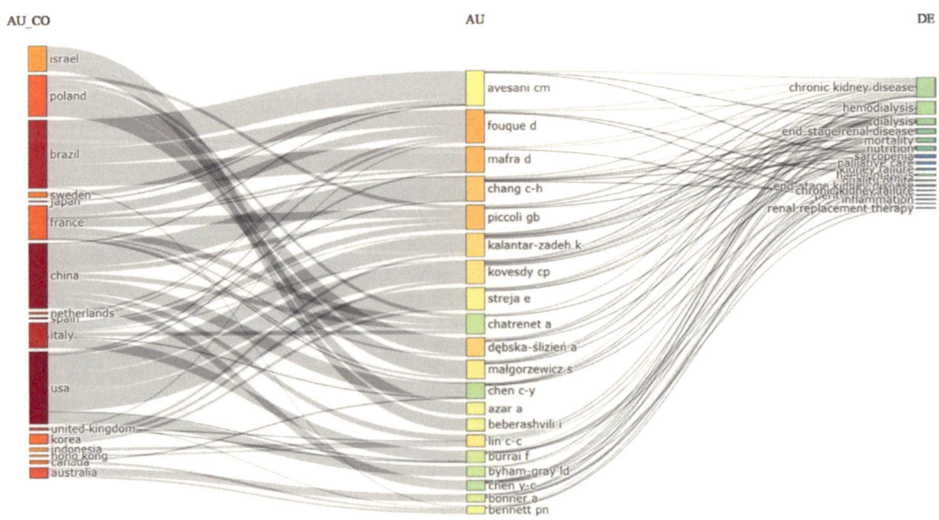

Figure 6.
Three-field diagram.

4.1.4 Three-field diagram

In this *Three-Field Diagram* layout, the program specifies three factors to be linked (country, author, and keyword), and **Figure 6** displays the most relevant items for each factor.

Also known as a Sankey diagram, this three-field diagram examines three parameters. According to the diagram, the importance of each parameter is indicated by the size of the rectangles.

In the diagram analyzing the parameters of country, author, and keyword, the most important country is the United States, the most prominent author is Fouque, and the most significant keyword is *chronic kidney disease*.

4.1.5 Most published journals

Between 2014 and 2025, based on the analysis using the keywords "hemodialysis," "art therapy," and "chronic kidney failure," *Journal of Renal Nutrition* ranked first with 62 articles, *Nutrients* ranked second with 44 articles, and *Journal of Renal Care* ranked third with 36 articles (**Table 3**).

4.1.6 Most productive authors

Table 4 lists the most influential authors worldwide in terms of publications.

Between 2014 and 2025, based on the analysis using the keywords "hemodialysis," "art therapy," and "chronic kidney failure," Fouque ranked first with seven publications, Mafra and Piccoli ranked second with five publications each, and Chang ranked third with four publications.

4.1.7 Most productive universities

Table 5 lists the institutions with the highest number of publications worldwide.

In the search using the keywords "Hemodialysis," "Art Therapy," and "Chronic Kidney Failure,"

Journals	Articles No
Journal of Renal Nutrition	62
Nutrients	44
Journal of Renal Care	36
Journal of Pain and Symptom Management	20
Clinical Nutrition Espen	12
Nutrients	11
Journal of Clinical Nursing	10
Journal of Palliative Medicine	9
Clinical Nutrition	7
Annals of Palliative Medicine	5

Table 3.
Most important journals.

Authors	Articles	Articles fractionalized
Fouque D	7	0,98
Mafra D	5	0,69
Piccoli Gb	5	0,94
Chang C-H	4	0,42
Dębska-Ślizień A	4	0,60
Kalantar-Zadeh K	4	0,53
Kovesdy Cp	4	0,53
Lin C-C	4	0,98
Małgorzewicz S	4	0,60
Streja E	4	0,62

Table 4.
Most productive authors.

Affiliation	Articles
Mayo Clinic	27
Osaka Metropolitan University Graduate School of Medicine	25
Fluminense Federal University (Uff)	18
Catholic University of Brasilia	17
Kidney Research Center	16
Medical University of Gdansk	16
Rutgers University	15
University of Pennsylvania	15
Kermanshah University of Medical Sciences	14
Leiden University Medical Center	14

Table 5.
Most productive universities.

- Mayo Clinic ranks first with 27 articles.
- Osaka Metropolitan University Graduate School of Medicine ranks second with 25 articles.
- Fluminense Federal University ranks third with 18 articles.

4.1.8 Most productive countries

Figure 7 shows the countries with the highest number of publications and citations based on the analysis of studies using the keywords "Hemodialysis," "Art Therapy," and "Chronic Kidney Failure." The map displays countries with the most publications, countries with the fewest publications, and countries with no publications at all.

The analysis of studies using the keywords "Hemodialysis," "Art Therapy," and "Chronic Kidney Failure" is presented on the world map in **Figure 7**, showing the most productive countries. On the map, the darkest color (navy blue) represents the country with the highest number of studies, blue and its shades indicate countries

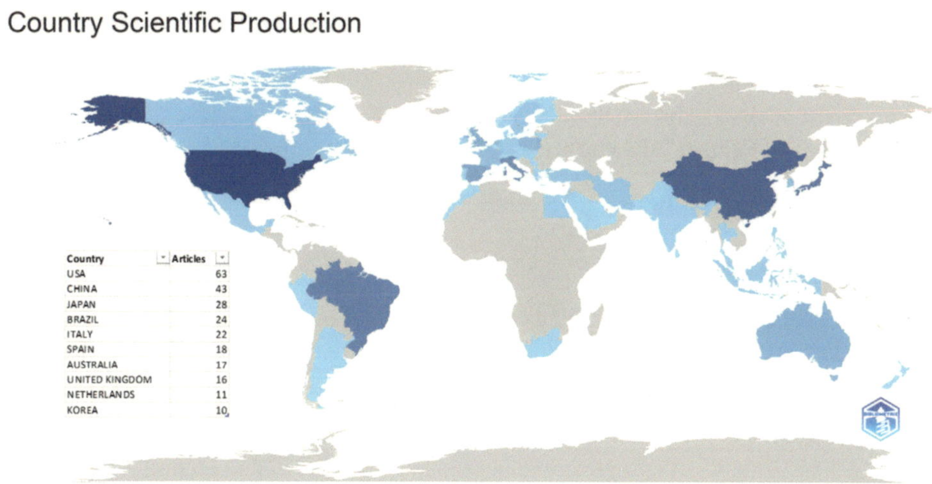

Figure 7.
Most productive countries.

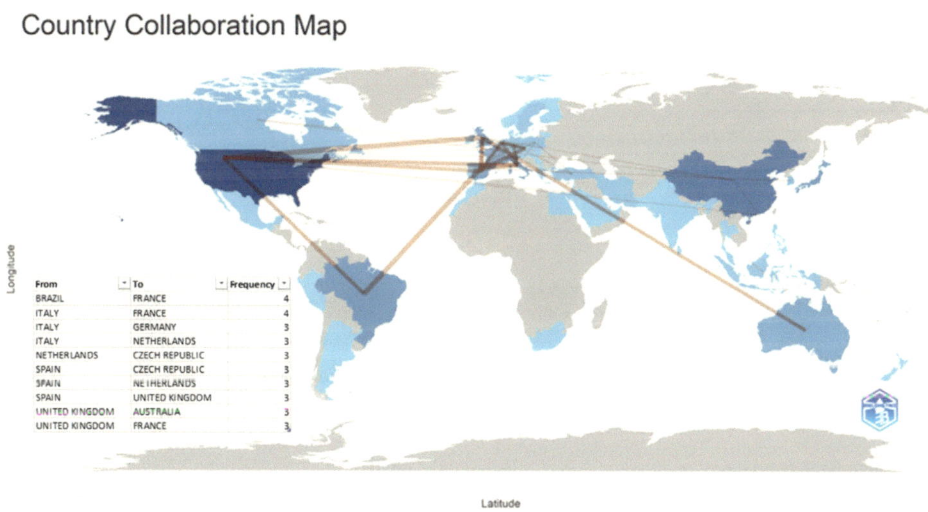

Figure 8.
Countries collaboration map.

with some publications, while gray indicates countries with no publications [13]. In the ranking of the most productive countries, the USA ranks first with 63 articles, China second with 43 articles, and Japan third with 28 articles.

Figure 8 shows the collaboration map between countries. According to the map, thick brown lines indicate a high number of collaborations between countries, while thin brown lines represent fewer collaborations. The term "countries collaboration map" refers to a visualization created by programs such as Biblioshiny to display scientific research collaborations between different countries. Such a map can be used to illustrate partnerships between researchers or institutions across countries for academic research purposes. The countries' collaboration map typically uses a network-based visualization method to present the level of collaboration between countries. Relationships between countries are shown with brown lines.

Brazil and France lead with four collaborations each, as do Italy and France with four collaborations. Brazil, France, and Italy are the leading countries in terms of collaboration (**Table 6**).

As a result of the analysis using the keywords "Hemodialysis," "Art Therapy," and "Chronic Kidney Failure," the countries with the highest number of citations are:

- The United States is in first place with 835 citations.
- Italy is in second place with 644 citations.
- Brazil is in third place with 390 citations.

Country	Total citations
The United States	835
Italy	644
Brazil	390
China	309
Spain	282
Australia	219
Israel	206
Japan	206
Netherlands	192
Iran	168

Table 6.
Most cited countries.

Paper	DOI	Total Citations
Cupıstı A, 2018, Nutrients	10.3390/Nu10030261	146
Borges Na, 2018, J Renal Nutr	10.1053/J.Jrn.2017.06.010	114
Noce A, 2019, Nutrients	10.3390/Nu11051073	113
Hmwe Ntt, 2015, Int J Nurs Stud	10.1016/J.İjnurstu.2014.11.002	113
Beberashvılı I, 2014, Eur J Clin Nutr	10.1038/Ejcn.2014.67	112
Rıbeıro Hs, 2022, Clin Nutr	10.1016/J.Clnu.2022.03.025	84
Luıs D, 2016, J Renal Nutr	10.1053/J.Jrn.2015.11.004	84
Bossola M, 2015, J Pain Symptom Manage	10.1016/J.Jpainsymman.2014.07.009	81
Tomayko Ej, 2015, J Renal Nutr	10.1053/J.Jrn.2014.10.005	76
Smyth A, 2016, J Renal Nutr	10.1053/J.Jrn.2016.01.016	74

Table 7.
Most cited publications.

4.1.9 Most cited publications

The most productive article is the one that has received the most citations. Consequently, **Table 7** presents the top 10 most productive articles based on the analysis using the keywords "Hemodialysis," "Art Therapy," and "Chronic Kidney Failure."

- Cupisti A et al.: Their 2018 article titled *"Dietary Approach to Recurrent or Chronic Hyperkalemia in Patients with Decreased Kidney Function,"* published in the journal *Nutrients*, ranks first with 146 citations.
- Borges NA et al.: Their 2018 article titled *"Probiotic Supplementation in Chronic Kidney Disease: A Double-blind, Randomized, Placebo-controlled Trial,"* published in *Randomized Controlled Trial*, ranks second with 114 citations.
- Noce A et al.: Their 2014 article titled *"Impact of Gut Microbiota Composition on Onset and Progression of Chronic Non-communicable Diseases,"* published in *Nutrients*, ranks third with 113 citations.

4.2 Analysis of scientific mapping

Scientific mapping uses computer tools to visualize, analyze, and simulate various scientific and technological processes. This method helps researchers better understand relationships, patterns, and trends within large datasets. Scientific mapping typically visually reveals relationships between texts, similarities or differences between topics, publication trends, and the significance of key concepts [13].

In this section, factor analysis, topic dendrogram, network map, and theme map based on author keywords are presented. These maps are used to visualize the conceptual structure of the research. They deepen the analysis and help understand conceptual connections within the study.

4.2.1 Factor analysis

Factor analysis is a statistical technique included in these tools, commonly used to reduce complexity and uncover latent structures in multivariate datasets. It is a

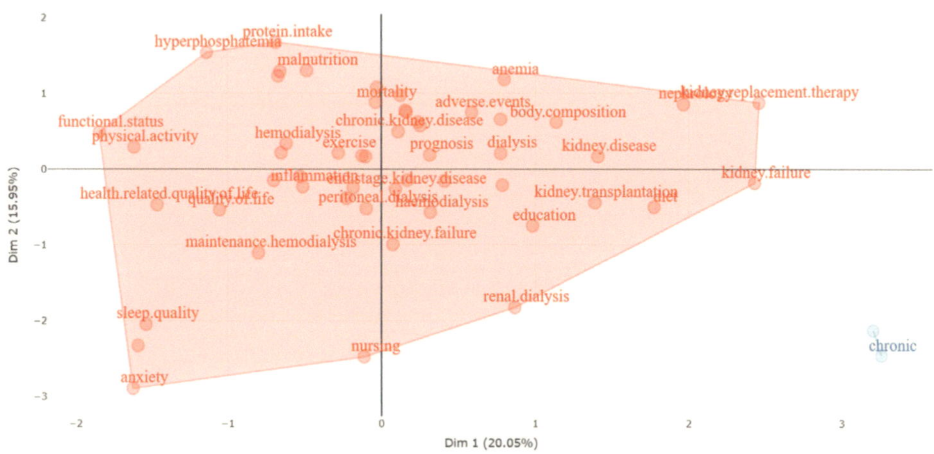

Figure 9.
Factor analysis of author keywords in articles using the keywords.

method used to understand relationships among variables in a dataset and to make the data more interpretable and manageable. This analysis is often expressed with coefficients called factor loadings, which indicate which factors are associated with variables or explain the commonality among specific variables [13]. The factor analysis created with keywords is shown in **Figure 9**.

"Hemodialysis," "Art Therapy," and "Chronic Kidney Failure". As a result of the factor analysis on the author keywords of the articles, it is observed that keywords such as *hemodialysis, chronic kidney disease, peritoneal dialysis, renal dialysis, anemia, and functional status* cluster together in the pink group.

4.2.2 Thematic map

Figure 10 shows a thematic map divided into four regions.

- The *motor themes* section of the diagram includes clusters representing the most fundamental research areas related to the keyword studied.

- The *basic themes* section includes clusters that represent core and evolving themes, meaning these are developing areas of study related to the keyword.

- The *emerging or declining themes* section shows newly emerging or fading keywords.

- The *niche themes* section indicates keywords with many studies, but those studies are isolated from others.

Therefore, to understand which scientific themes are prominent for the given keywords, it is important to focus on the basic and motor theme sections of the

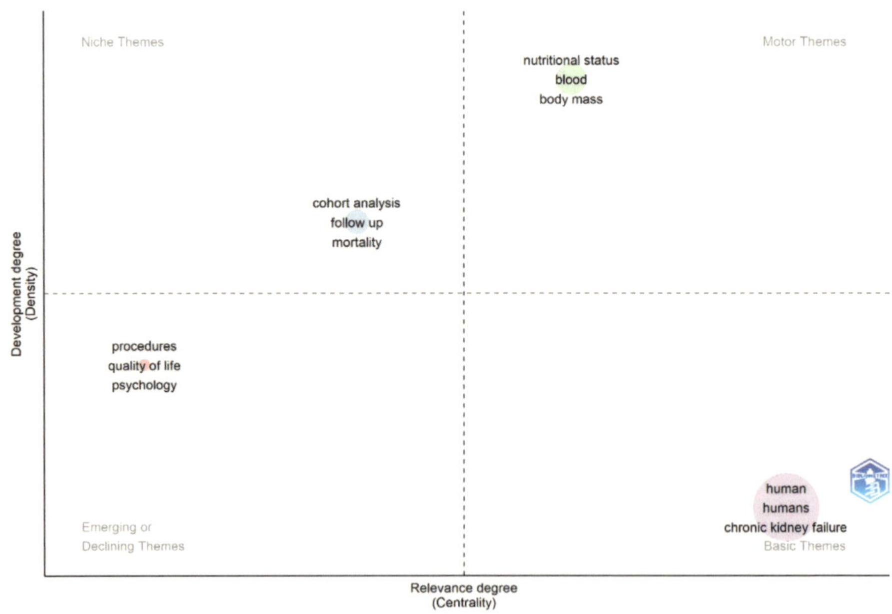

Figure 10.
Thematic map.

diagram [13]. **Figure 10** demonstrates that the studies cluster under two main themes with varying intensities.

In the motor theme cluster, the keywords nutritional status, blood, and body mass are observed.

For the niche theme, the keywords include cohort analysis, follow-up, and mortality. The emerging or declining theme contains procedures, quality of life, and psychology. In the basic theme, the keywords human, humans, and chronic kidney failure are found.

4.2.3 Trending topics

Table 8 presents the trending topics in the literature by year from 2014 to 2025.

- The term *"Renal replacement therapy"* appeared 118 times and was the most popular term in the first quarter of 2015, the second quarter of 2017, and the third quarter of 2020.
- The term *"Art therapy"* appeared 24 times and was popular in the first quarter of 2014, the second quarter of 2015, and the third quarter of 2018.
- The term *"United States"* appeared 16 times and was popular in the first quarter of 2014, the second quarter of 2016, and the third quarter of 2019.

4.2.4 Keyword analysis

A keyword is a term or phrase used to describe an article. The presence of a keyword in an article affects the frequency of that expression [13]. To highlight the typical results of the study with keywords and the research database, VOSviewer 1.6.20 was used.

Figure 11 illustrates the keywords and their clustering patterns. The keywords have formed 16 different clusters. Based on the size of the clusters, the most important keywords are *hemodialysis* (highlighted in yellow), *chronic kidney disease* (dark blue), and *hemodialysis* (light blue).

Table 9 provides a summary of the main types of interventions in hemodialysis. Accordingly, dietary management, psychosocial support, medication management, patient education, physical activity, spiritual care, and technological innovations were

Term	Frequency	Year (Q1)	Year (median)	Year (Q3)
Adverse effects	10	2014	2014	2015
Europe	10	2014	2014	2016
Questionnaires	6	2014	2014	2015
Art therapy	24	2014	2015	2018
Phosphate intake	14	2014	2015	2017
Phosphorus, dietary	9	2014	2015	2017
The United States	16	2014	2016	2019
Dietary proteins	15	2014	2016	2018
Follow-up studies	13	2015	2016	2020
Renal replacement therapy	118	2015	2017	2020

Table 8.
Trending topics.

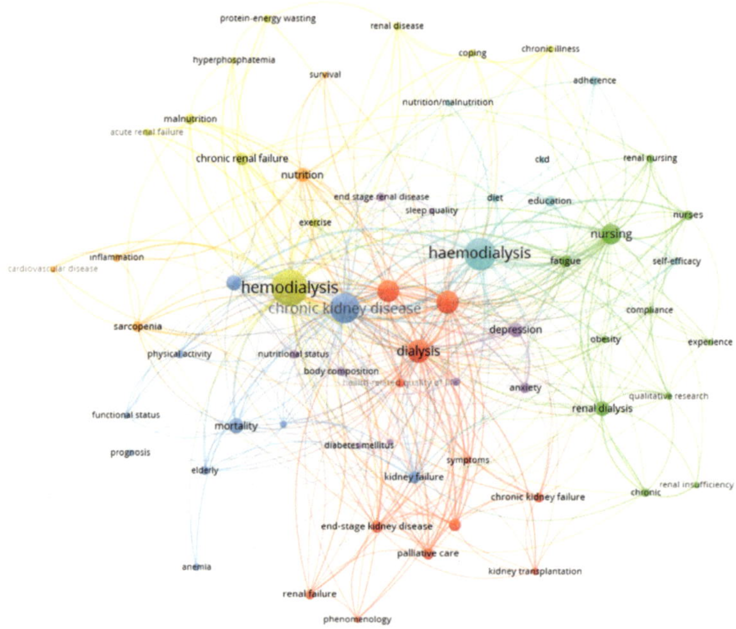

Figure 11.
Keyword network map.

Intervention type	Description	Impact on quality of life
Dietary management	Individualized dietary plans for potassium, phosphate, and fluid control	Improves physical well-being and symptom control
Psychosocial support	Counseling, support groups, and psychiatric care	Enhances emotional well-being and coping capacity
Medication management	Adherence to phosphate binders, antihypertensives, and erythropoietin	Improves symptom control and biochemical parameters
Patient education	Training on a visual table summarizing those interventions as mentioned: dialysis procedures, hygiene, and symptom monitoring	Promotes self-efficacy and treatment adherence
Physical activity	Supervised exercise programs during or between sessions	Improves physical function and reduces fatigue
Spiritual care	Integration of cultural/religious practices and chaplaincy support	Improves resilience and life satisfaction
Technological innovations	Use of smart devices, wearable monitoring, and telehealth	Facilitates monitoring and personalized care

Table 9.
Summary of the main types of interventions in hemodialysis [1, 3, 9, 10].

identified as the key intervention types for hemodialysis patients. The impact of these intervention types on the quality of life of hemodialysis patients is shown in **Table 9**.

In the timeline of keywords shown in **Figure 12**, the dark blue colors represent keywords that have been studied and completed in the literature, such as *art therapy*, *hemodialysis*, and *chronic renal failure* during the years 2010–2012.

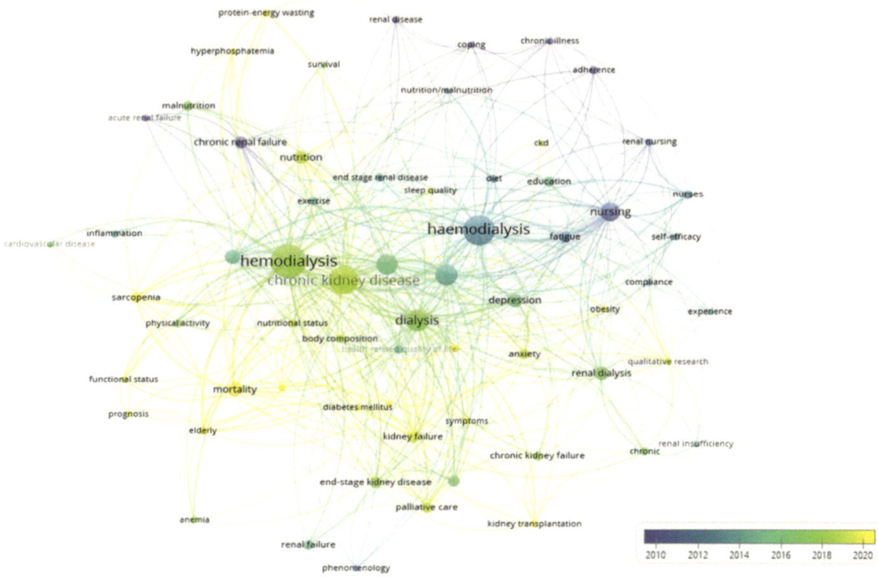

Figure 12.
Timeline of keywords.

Green and its shades correspond to the period between 2016 and 2018, highlighting keywords like *hemodialysis*, *dialysis*, and *renal dialysis*.

The yellow colors on the timeline indicate keywords that are still actively studied in the literature, including *mortality*, *symptoms*, *kidney failure*, *kidney transplantation*, *anxiety*, and *obesity* (**Figure 13**).

In the word cloud, the most frequently repeated words are *hemodialysis, female*, and *chronic kidney failure* (**Figure 14**).

In the tree map, the size of the rectangles represents how frequently the words are used. The words *male* and *female* appear most frequently, each accounting for 8% of occurrences and ranking first. The words *aged* and *middle-aged* follow with a frequency of 6%, ranking

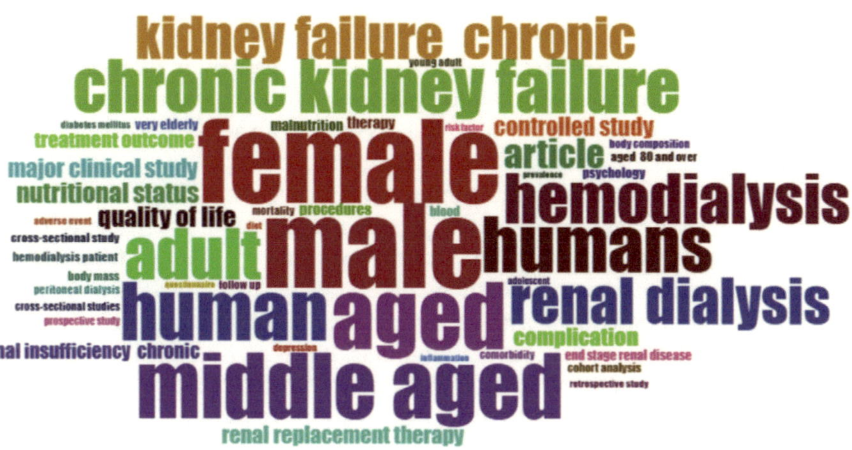

Figure 13.
Word cloud.

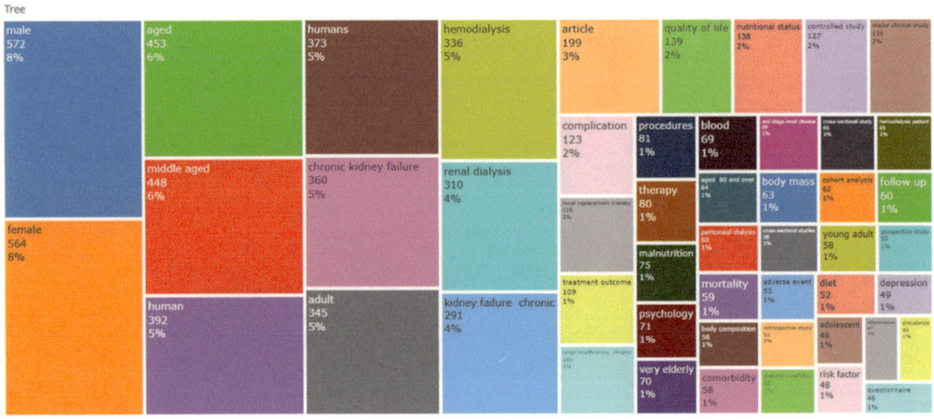

Figure 14.
Tree map.

second. The words *human*, *humans*, *chronic kidney failure*, *adult*, and *hemodialysis* each occur with a frequency of 5%, making up the top three frequently repeated keywords.

5. Discussion

The theoretical explanations underlying the effectiveness of art therapy in hemodialysis patients can be interpreted through psychodynamic, cognitive-behavioral, humanistic, and neurobiological frameworks. From a psychodynamic perspective, the art process allows the symbolic expression of unconscious conflicts, fears, and anger related to the illness. Visual images represent feelings that are difficult to verbalize, aiding insight development. From a cognitive-behavioral viewpoint, art therapy provides tools for recognizing and restructuring negative automatic thoughts. Patients can question negative schemas associated with their "patient" identity. The humanistic approach supports self-expression, choice, and meaning-making in life. Art products enhance patients' sense of self-efficacy.

At the neurobiological level, creative activities are proposed to modulate limbic system activity, reduce stress responses, and stimulate dopamine and endorphin release [9, 19]. These theoretical models are especially relevant in dialysis, as dialysis sessions are passive processes that require patients to be connected to a machine for hours. Art therapy invites patients out of passivity into an active creative process, enhancing self-efficacy that supports treatment adherence.

Research highlights practical advantages of art therapy in dialysis centers. The long hours during dialysis are often boring and tiring for patients. Art activities make this time meaningful and "productive." Art therapy may positively influence treatment continuation rates and appointment adherence [8, 10]. It offers opportunities to build new narratives for coping with chronic illness identity. Patients can identify not only as "patients" but also as creative individuals. It fosters new collaboration models among dialysis nurses, nephrologists, psychologists, and art therapists. Such holistic approaches align with the World Health Organization's integrated chronic disease management model [20].

Although art therapy in hemodialysis patients has been found to moderately reduce depression and anxiety levels, improve quality of life, and increase patient satisfaction, important limitations affect the interpretation of these findings: most studies have small sample sizes (10–30 participants), randomized controlled trials (RCTs) are limited, and many are pilot or pre–post test designs. Intervention durations (4–12 weeks), session frequencies (one to two times per week), and implementation content (painting, collage, and storytelling) are heterogeneous. Different psychological scales reduce comparability of results. Most studies measure short-term effects; long-term sustainability is unknown. This methodological heterogeneity hinders meta-analyses and limits clinical guideline development [21–28].

While art therapy offers a universal framework, cultural norms, esthetic understandings, and modes of expression vary across societies. For example, in South Korea, due to community-focused and hierarchical relationships, sharing emotions in groups requires special structuring [9]. Studies in Chile show Catholic symbolism, themes of hope, and forgiveness reflected in artistic products [8]. Qualitative theses from Turkey (YÖK Thesis Center data) have begun examining the relationship between individual/group art therapy, perceptions of privacy, and cultural sensitivities. In this context, it is recommended that art therapy protocols be culturally sensitive and allow patients space for symbolic expression.

Cultural factors, including elements such as language, religion, tradition, family structure, and social norms that shape individuals' beliefs, attitudes, behaviors, and health-related decision-making, have both direct and indirect effects on the quality of life of hemodialysis patients [29]. Because they play a decisive role in the success of hemodialysis treatment, cultural factors are vital for providing culturally sensitive healthcare, increasing patient compliance, and improving quality of life. Different cultures influence not only medical interventions but also individual disease perception, treatment adherence, and quality of life in hemodialysis patients. For example, disease perception varies across cultures. Some societies view illness as fate, while others associate it with individual responsibility. This perspective influences patient compliance with treatment, adherence to dietary guidelines, and coping skills [30]. Religious rituals such as fasting can influence hemodialysis programs. For example, in Hindu and Buddhist societies, some patients may prefer traditional healers or Ayurvedic practices over medical treatment. In Muslim societies, the desire to fast during Ramadan may lead patients to restrict fluid intake and skip dialysis sessions. Thirty-eight percent of HD patients in Saudi Arabia spend Ramadan [31]. All these cultural factors necessitate healthcare professionals to develop personalized care plans that take cultural factors into account. Future studies are recommended to more comprehensively examine the impact of culture on quality of life through cross-cultural comparisons.

The literature search [e.g., Web of Science/Scopus] identified 402 articles from 118 journals indexed in Scopus between 2014 and 2025 on hemodialysis and art therapy. The annual distribution of studies using the keywords "hemodialysis," "art therapy," and "chronic kidney failure" showed 28 studies in 2023, 63 in 2024, and 38 in 2025, with the highest publication number in 2024. These results indicate a relatively emerging research area bridging medical, art, psychological, and public health disciplines.

As art therapy becomes more visible in general medicine, its adoption in nephrology has increased. The greater emphasis on psychosocial support needs in clinical guidelines for chronic patients plays a role in this growth.

The total citations per article were 0.61 in 2025, 1.68 in 2024, and 4.54 in 2023. The overall citation volume remains low, reflecting limited research activity. However, the citation curve shows growing interdisciplinary interest, with psychiatry, nephrology, and psychology fields citing the literature.

In diagrams examining country, author, and keyword parameters, the United States is the most significant country, Fouque the key author, and "chronic kidney disease" the most important keyword. The 2014 three-field plot shows the topic appearing in nutrition-focused journals such as *Journal of Renal Nutrition*, as well as multidisciplinary care journals like *Journal of Renal Care*, highlighting its interdisciplinary nature.

The field mostly develops within nutrition and psychosocial care journals, with limited presence in pure medical nephrology journals. Author analysis reveals a few small leading research teams but limited large-scale international networks, which restrict the integration of the topic into global guidelines. Applications aimed at psychosocial support through art therapy are more commonly reported in Western countries. Although there has been recent momentum in countries like Turkey, publication numbers remain low. Strengthening collaboration networks is recommended. Citation intensity tends to focus on methodologically robust and clinically applicable intervention studies, motivating well-designed RCTs in the future.

This bibliometric analysis shows that the theme of art therapy and hemodialysis is a developing research area with increasing publication and citation trends, but still has a limited and regionally concentrated volume. In this context, further art therapy studies, strengthening international collaborations, and integration of psychosocial interventions into nephrology guidelines are recommended.

Hemodialysis treatment is a process of high clinical complexity, requiring multidisciplinary approaches. Bibliometric findings indicate that most publications are biomedically based, but there is a relative lack of applied studies directly impacting clinical decision-making processes. Instead of currently standardized hemodialysis protocols, personalized treatments tailored to patient characteristics are necessary to reduce mortality and morbidity rates. Therefore, studies on individualized dialysis durations and frequencies, taking into account genetics, biomarkers, and patient-reported outcome measures (PROMs), should be a topic of future research [32, 33]. The prevalence of depression, anxiety, and social isolation in long-term hemodialysis patients negatively impacts treatment adherence and overall prognosis. Therefore, prospective studies are crucial for future research, particularly integrating structured psychosocial support programs into clinical practice. In addition to the physiological effects of hemodialysis treatment, the impact of integrated treatment methods, particularly art therapy, on patients' psychosocial status, depression, anxiety, and social life should be considered, and multidisciplinary studies focusing on quality of life should be prioritized. Future research directions, focusing on clinical practice in hemodialysis patients, should be shaped by interdisciplinary approaches to both improve patients' quality of life and improve treatment outcomes.

In other words, increasing treatment effectiveness, reducing complications, and improving the quality of life of hemodialysis patients should be considered the primary goals of future research. With this understanding, it is crucial to comprehensively evaluate individualized treatment strategies, new technological integrations, innovative dialysis approaches, and psychosocial support systems and rapidly implement them into clinical practice. To ensure success and sustainable benefits in clinical practice, conducting research within a multidisciplinary approach will not only strengthen clinical practice in hemodialysis but also directly contribute to the overall quality of life of patients.

The current literature signals a promising yet evolving field. First, randomized controlled trials are scarce; larger samples and well-defined protocols are needed. Second, long-term follow-up is lacking; effects beyond 6 months to 1 year are unknown. Third, culturally sensitive intervention designs are limited; art therapy should be adapted to each society's symbolic language. Fourth, cost-effectiveness analyses are missing; economic arguments are necessary to secure health policy funding for such supportive services [34]. Finally, increasing qualitative research is advised. Patient experiences, narratives, and themes from art products can make service design more meaningful.

Bibliometric analyses examine not only the temporal and geographical distribution of research outputs but also the evolution of thematic priorities such as psychosocial interventions, technological innovations, and patient education. While the study effectively maps publication trends, **Table 8**, which summarizes key intervention types, can enrich the applied perspective and provide a more comprehensive understanding of clinical applications. This perspective supports healthcare providers, including healthcare professionals and interdisciplinary teams, in translating research findings into practical strategies. Furthermore, this approach will lead to the integration of content analyses of interventions reported in high-impact publications in future studies, further strengthening the practical applicability of bibliometric findings.

In conclusion, while art therapy emerges as a promising intervention for depression, anxiety, and quality of life in hemodialysis patients, academic production in the field remains insufficient. Bibliometric analysis offers valuable insights for researchers in strategic planning, collaboration development, and identifying gaps in the literature.

Author details

Songül Mollaoğlu[1] and Mukadder Mollaoğlu[2*]

1 Faculty of Education, Department of Fine Arts Education, Sivas Cumhuriyet University, Sivas, Turkey

2 Faculty of Health Sciences, Sivas Cumhuriyet University, Sivas, Turkey

*Address all correspondence to: mollaoglumukadder@gmail.com

References

[1] Bikbov B, Purcell CA, Levey AS, Smith M, Abdoli A, Abebe M, et al. Global, regional, and national burden of chronic kidney disease, 1990-2017: A systematic analysis for the global burden of disease study 2017. Lancet. 2020;**395**(10225):709-733

[2] Barbar SD, Bourredjem A, Trusson R, Dargent A, Binquet C, Quenot JP, et al. Differential effect on mortality of the timing of initiation of renal replacement therapy according to the criteria used to diagnose acute kidney injury: An IDEAL-ICU substudy. Critical Care. 2023;**27**(1):316

[3] Palmer S, Vecchio M, Craig JC, Tonelli M, Johnson DW, Nicolucci A, et al. Prevalence of depression in chronic kidney disease: Systematic review and meta-analysis of observational studies. Kidney International. 2013;**84**(1):179-191

[4] Chilcot J, Davenport A, Wellsted D. An association between depressive symptoms and survival in incident dialysis patients. Nephrology, Dialysis, Transplantation. 2011;**26**(5):1628-1634

[5] Lopes AA, Bragg J, Young E, Goodkin D, Mapes D, Combe C, et al. Depression as a predictor of mortality and hospitalization among hemodialysis patients in the United States and Europe. Kidney International. 2002;**62**(1):199-207

[6] Malchiodi CA. Handbook of Art Therapy. 3rd ed. New York: Guilford Press; 2003. pp. 431-448

[7] Garcia-Diaz. The effect of the practice of Authentic Movement on the emotional state. Arts in Psychotherapy. 2018;**58**:17-26. DOI: 10.1016/j.aip.2018.03.004

[8] Huss E. Havsteen-franklin D. Developing a theory of social art therapy: Insights from the context of crisis. Arts in Psychotherapy. 2023;**85**:102066

[9] Wang Y, Yang L, Lei Y. The global status of nursing research on hemodialysis: A bibliometric and visualized analysis. Medicine (Baltimore). 27 Sep 2024;**103**(39):e39707. DOI: 10.1097/MD.0000000000039707

[10] Mollaoğlu M, Candan F, Solmaz G, Mollaoğlu S, Başer E, Yanmiş S. The effect of education and art therapy with telehealth method on diet-fluid restriction and anxiety in hemodialysis patients during the Covid-19 pandemic. Alternative Therapies in Health and Medicine. 2024 Jul;**30**(7):58-64

[11] Ritianingsih N, Nurhayati F, Salmid A. Art therapy on stress and anxiety of chronic kidney failure (crf) patients with hemodialysis in Bogor City Hospital. Indonesian Journal of Health Sciences Research and Development. 2022;**4**(3):527-534

[12] Ruhanen L, Weiler B, Moyle B, McLennan C. Trends and patterns in sustainable tourism research: A 25 year bibliometric analysis. Journal of Sustainable Tourism. 2015;**23**(4):517-535

[13] Demir G, Chatterjee P, Zakeri S, Pamucar D. Mapping the evolution of multi-attributive border approximation area comparison method: A bibliometric analysis. Decision Making: Applications in Management and Engineering. 2024;**7**(1):290-314

[14] Bashar A, Singh S, Pathak VK. A bibliometric review of online impulse buying behavior literature. International

Journal of Electronic Business. 2022;**17**(2):162-183

[15] Hassan MK, Rabbani MR, Brodmann J, et al. Bibliometric and scientometric analysis on CSR practices in the banking sector. Review of Financial Economics. 2022;**41**(2):177-196

[16] Ferreira FGDC, Gandomi AH, Cardoso RTN. Artificial intelligence applied to stock market trading: A review. IEEE Access. 2021;**9**:30898-30917

[17] Haque MI, Ahmad S, Azad MS. Mapping of scientific literature on Islamic Economics, Banking and Finance 1955 to 2020. Library Philosophy and Practice (e-journal). 2020:4306. Available from: https://digitalcommons.unl.edu/libphilprac/4306

[18] Aria M, Cuccurullo C. Bibliometrix: An R-tool for comprehensive science mapping analysis. Journal of Informetrics. 2017;**11**(4):959-975

[19] Kaimal G, Walker MS, Herres J, Deaver SP. Art therapy for psychological and somatic symptoms associated with medical conditions. In: Malchiodi CA, editor. Handbook of Art Therapy. 3rd ed. New York: Guilford Press; 2003. pp. 431-448

[20] World Health Organization. Noncommunicable diseases: Key facts. 2020. Available from: https://www.who.int/news-room/fact-sheets/detail/noncommunicable-diseases

[21] Liu Z, Yang Z, Xiao C, Zhang K, Osmani M. An investigation into art therapy aided health and well-being research: A 75-year bibliometric analysis. International Journal of Environmental Research and Public Health. 2021;**19**(1):232

[22] Rodriguez Novo N, Novo Muñoz MM, Cuellar-Pompa L, Rodriguez Gomez JA. Trends in research on art therapy indexed in the web of science: A bibliometric analysis. Frontiers in Psychology. 2021;**12**:752026. DOI: 10.3389/fpsyg.2021.752026

[23] Wu JF, Chung CY. Art therapy as an intervention for children: A bibliometric analysis of publications from 1990 to 2020. SAGE Open. 2023;**13**(4):1-16

[24] Lopez-Escribano C, Orío-Aparicio C, Lopez M, Cao F. An overview of historical and contemporary perspectives in art therapy in Spain: A bibliometric analysis of Spanish art therapy research. The Arts in Psychotherapy. 2023;**83**:10201

[25] Wang JH, Abdullah AB. A summary of expressive arts therapy and painting therapy. Creative Education. 2024;**15**:278-288

[26] Sun Z, Chen Z, Liu R, Lu G, Li Z, Sun Y. Research progress on the efficacy and safety of spironolactone in reversing left ventricular hypertrophy in hemodialysis patients. Drug Design, Development and Therapy. 2023 Jan;**23**(17):181-190

[27] Lee HJ, Kim HJ, Kim SY, Choi H. A study on how art therapy affect the depression, anxiety, stress, and satisfaction experienced by immigrant "Koryo-saram" adolescents. Korean Journal of Art Therapy. 2021;**28**(3):659-672

[28] Kresnowati L, Suhartono S, Shaluhiyah Z, Widjanarko B. Finding the new potential research on diabetic kidney disease and hemodialysis in healthcare insurance databases: A bibliometric analysis. Narra J. 2024 Dec;**4**(3):e827

[29] Yonata A, Islamy N, Taruna A, Pura L. Factors Affecting Quality of Life

in Hemodialysis Patients. International Journal of General Medicine. 12 Sep 2022;**15**:7173-7178. DOI: 10.2147/IJGM.S375994

[30] Ashing-Giwa KT. The contextual model of health-related quality of life: Revisiting the theoretical foundation of HRQOL. Quality of Life Research. 2005;**14**(2):273-282

[31] Emara AA, Ghareeb AH, Fayez M, Elsharabasy RM. Ramadan fasting in hemodialysis population: Single-center study. Egyptian Journal of Internal Medicine. 2022;**34**(1):63. DOI: 10.1186/s43162-022-00150-8

[32] Devins GM, Mendelssohn DC, Barre PE, Binik YM. Predialysis psychoeducational intervention and coping styles influence time to dialysis in chronic kidney disease. American Journal of Kidney Diseases. 2003;**42**(4):693-703

[33] Pagels AA, Söderkvist BK, Medin C, Hylander B, Heiwe S. Health-related quality of life in different stages of chronic kidney disease and at initiation of dialysis treatment. Health and Quality of Life Outcomes. 2012;**10**:71

[34] Uttley L, Stevenson M, Scope A, Rawdin A, Taylor Buck E, Sutton A, et al. Systematic review and economic modelling of the clinical effectiveness and cost-effectiveness of art therapy among people with non-psychotic mental health disorders. Health Technology Assessment. 2015;**19**(18):1-120. DOI: 10.3310/hta19180

Section 2

Evidence-Based Approaches

Chapter 4

Exploring the Transformative Impact of Technology on Evidence-Based Healthcare

Elisabeta Shehu Kafia

Abstract

The use of modern information technologies by health practitioners in their evidence-based practice contributes to the improvement of the system and raises public confidence in healthcare services. It certainly supports society's goals of patient participation and independence, but it is of great importance that health professionals are comfortable using such advanced technologies. Using the right information technology is surely one of the best ways to achieve the findings that will make the difference between a good and indifferent practitioner.

Keywords: technology, evidence-based healthcare, data analytics, clinical decision support systems, artificial intelligence, digital health tools

1. Introduction

The ultimate mission of healthcare is to efficiently and powerfully alter or maintain human physiology to achieve optimal or maximum health. However, this is challenging considering the extremely complex nature of the human body and most health issues. It becomes immediately obvious that to meet these exigencies, healthcare outcomes should not only rely on robust evidence but also on technology that allows the most accurate organized information to be made easily accessible and shared. This chapter explores the intersections of evidence-based practice and information technology, discussing briefly the historical context, some current best practices and a summary of the impacts on society.

Now that knowledge has become more reliable and grounded in reason, evidence and causation, the concept of evidence-based practice has emerged. The earliest evidence-based practice example was "suicide prohibition at the British Army," in which they ordered the British soldiers not to have bullets in their guns when sleeping. Evidence-based medicine was nurtured at universities, where training programs for health professionals presented a new evidence-based medicine model. Most scholars consider that evidence-based medicine is nurtured from evidence-based practice, and both share agreements concerning evidence-based practice.

The transformative impact of technology on evidence-based healthcare is increasingly recognized as a vital component in enhancing the accessibility, quality and efficiency of health services. But careful consideration should be given to the complex role of digital health interventions and the associated challenges in their implementation and effectiveness.

As Erku et al. [1] highlight the dual nature of digital health interventions in primary healthcare, these technologies have the potential to improve access and delivery, particularly in underserved rural areas, but they also pose some significant ethical concerns regarding confidentiality and equitable access. The findings of this study underline that the adoption of telemedicine during the COVID-19 pandemic has not only transformed healthcare delivery but has also exacerbated existing inequalities, particularly affecting vulnerable populations.

Building on these insights, Mumtaz et al. [2] address the challenges and potential solutions in the use of digital health technologies for evidence generation. The authors argue that for digital healthcare technologies to be effectively integrated into clinical practice, a strong emphasis on evaluation through complex systems and evidence-based frameworks is essential. They highlight the importance of addressing ethical considerations, such as user consent and socioeconomic disparities, which are critical for ensuring equitable access to digital health benefits.

Building upon the findings of recent studies, this chapter illustrates the necessity of a balanced approach to the integration of technology in evidence-based healthcare, recognizing both the opportunities and challenges that digital health presents.

This chapter explores basic principles for using information technology more effectively in evidence-based care. It gives an overview of:

1. Why does evidence-based practice lead to better patient outcomes compared to other healthcare practices?

2. What kinds of information technology applications are most beneficial to healthcare, and what are their merits?

3. How each technology can be applied in evidence-based practice to improve patient outcomes?

Implementing modern information technologies in evidence-based healthcare providers builds public trust in the services and social objectives of patient involvement and autonomy. Health professionals need to be skilled in using such advanced technologies. The use of relevant information technology is undoubtedly among the most effective ways of obtaining insights that distinguish between an experienced practitioner and one who is not so skilled.

In the field of healthcare, evidence-based practice is an essential tool for enhancing the quality and safety of care provided to patients. It embodies "the best research evidence and agency for patients, as well as clinical and administrative expertise, and individual patient preferences" and is designed to offer a scientific basis upon which clinical decisions can be made.

1.1 Definitions and principles

Defining and guiding principles for research, tools and methodologies for producing scientifically sound information about the risk to human health are among the most important but least appreciated human achievements to date. These advances explain the dramatic increase in healthy life expectancy, world productivity and standards of living during the past century. The high cost and difficulty of obtaining specialist knowledge, tools and methodologies required to develop, produce and assure safe delivery and performance of medical technologies continue to challenge society, however. The highest quality of care for most people, consideration in policies and decision-making when resources are limited, and sustained improvements in health status and productivity require evidence-based common principles as the basis of medicine and the underlying medical technologies, systems and methodologies.

Evidence-based medicine promotes better care and healthcare systems by evaluating and using the best available research evidence and other evidence to support claims about the risks and benefits of care options. Translated into healthcare terms, it includes the efficacy and risk of the many medical technologies used in patient care. For most individual care decisions, the claims and choices that define the healthcare problem have to be applied to the best available scientific knowledge, probabilities and harms collected using research tools and treatment assessment methods appropriate to the problem and alternatives. The very specialized education and experience that should be required to develop, interpret and decide the validity and applicability of the specific care decision of the many different scientific disciplines and standards underpinning medical evidence is, however, the exception rather than the rule. This has led to the development of medical evidence in the form of inventions, discoveries or technology without commercial application for the care provider to help them obtain and evaluate, identify and interpret the determinants of what is relevant to the patient's characteristics and situation, and use the results of the best evidence for tending to the patient's healthcare problem.

1.2 Importance of information technology in healthcare

Rapid development, adoption and diffusion have changed the nature of healthcare. In healthcare, where IT is becoming a strategic asset and where huge government investments in systems have been realized, this is particularly relevant. Attempts to understand ethical, legal and social implications of health IT have mostly focused on issues facing healthcare providers and institutions. Yet IT is increasingly used to engage patients with their healthcare and medical data through electronic medical records, patient access systems, health apps and patient support networks. Doctor-patient relationships have changed because people are less willing to agree with decisions made by professionals who might not have their best interests at heart. With data readily available and easily analyzed, people have more access to information. It is led to greater citizen participation in decisions affecting their lives. Thus, the center of control is shifting more and more to the patient's hands.

But with this shift came many problems. The issue of trust in systems that collect data/present information/allow transactions/deliver therapies/interventions to the patient has become very important. And for people, this is their first line of defense—and trusting technology in the healthcare context is crucial. And people also feel that to get really involved with personal data and use it to make informed decisions, it takes an extension of one's identity or a leap of faith that the system is acting in their best interests.

A second issue is how much data is available. It is accepted that we are living in the information age, but processing data can be like finding a needle in a haystack. Systems that can use data for appropriate analyses, which protect personal data, and which simultaneously harvest the most important data features for better decisions are not always on the shelves.

Lastly, the explosion of health-related data harvested by both private and government systems creates new questions and issues regarding who owns our data and who is authorized to use it. Individuals feel that they have the exclusive right to control access and usage. That set off a national and then a global debate on laws that protect individuals' data and give them a share in the benefits of manipulating personalized knowledge bases.

2. Role of technology in healthcare

Technology can be transformative, but the healthcare challenge is about people—doctors, nurses, patients and carers. Technologies allow these healthcare actors to do tasks and play work/personal roles. Technology should improve patient care—including the care experience. The technology benefits should not stop at the task and check level since the system is concerned with evidence input, clinical task processing and decision output. Technology should support professional clinical decision-making and not be prescriptive in providing healthcare. Technologies may be subtle, as clinical consultations will remain the main mode of delivery for healthcare. But technology in healthcare is valuable and opens windows of opportunity to break open systems and re-engineer care.

Healthcare is a system. Introduction and configuration of health information technologies may induce change on many levels. Some are predictable, and others are not expected. Sociotechnical explanations of such mixed outcomes are given below. Relationships between healthcare staff, information systems and medical knowledge technology systems create the conditions for such technology-enabled healthcare. Positive opportunities include making invisible evidence visible, ensuring relevant evidence will be found automatically, ensuring timely provision of evidence for decision-making and personalizing evidence for each patient. This is not just clinical information but implicit patient evidence that the patient is healthy, that care is provided, and that caring will guide patient management decisions. The hidden connotations behind the evidence have social and economic consequences for the patient and healthcare stakeholders. Designs and deployments of health technology enable evidence from the healthcare process to be captured and used in ways never before possible—this will drive process evolution in healthcare. Other known negative outcomes and potential unwanted consequences need to be minimized as well. These might include unsynchronization of work processes and clinical information sequences, medical errors, over-utilization of technology, constant change demands, inappropriate data access and use, inadequate privacy and confidentiality protection and lack of proper care practices [1]. Healthcare IT implementations should therefore be viewed as interrupters of unsafe organizational and clinical behavior patterns. Organizations have to modify processes and systems to accommodate and promote the proper use of such support tools. Optimizing the usage of implemented systems is important and sharing lessons learned will benefit other similar organizations.

2.1 Overview of technological advancements

Technology is constantly being renovated and healthcare may be the most immediate example of this transformative nature of technological advancements. Although technology is often at the top of solutions for universal healthcare delivery in modernized countries, we have seen that technology is not sufficient. Yet, equality and better care delivery models for healthcare will always require technology in some form—whether telemedicine to mobilize scarce resources across remote reaches of care delivery, smart home care systems testing basic vital signs as early indicators or patient access systems enabling self-care at home to avoid readmissions.

Tech-enabled care expansion has broad political support; indeed, one survey found that many respondents listed the following as a benefit of digital technologies: Remote monitoring, advice and support are possible [2]. Other than providing healthcare without unnecessary movements, digital health applications can help with health management. They both allow the extraction of meaningful health data, improve patient health and contribute to prevention. Information derived from the technologies we create can improve healthcare and processes for curing diseases or maintaining health because it puts evidence into practice for patients being treated—evidence-based practice.

2.2 Benefits and challenges

Information technology is the set of tools, resources and technological access required for the capture, storage, transmission, transformation and use of health information. IT should position the consumer and health professional as partners in acquiring, including, discussing and assessing healthcare quality, safety and effectiveness. In this respect, IT redefines health knowledge. They give the clinician access to newer clinical information technologies for rational clinical decision making and healthcare effectiveness.

For evidence-based practice, a broader view might be useful—one that integrates questions formulation, evidence identification, review and appraisal, dissemination of results, application and evaluation of results and context in which they are applied. Integration of IT in a national healthcare system will optimize the application of scientific knowledge on clinical efficacy, as well as prevent and manage diseases, improve healthcare social processes of quality, efficiency and equity and transform market incentives of the health system by linking the individual health decision-making process [3].

3. Integration of technology in evidence-based healthcare

The integration of technology in evidence-based healthcare has enabled dramatic changes in virtually all areas of humanity. Healthcare is one of the areas where biotechnology has made significant contributions. In evidence-based practice, technology has supported many changes in prevention, diagnosis, treatment and monitoring. In a matter of seconds, healthcare professionals can get the latest evidence from the Internet anywhere and anytime. This fast access to systematically evaluated information at the point of care is a new form of knowledge management.

Given our rapidly changing society and the explosion of information about health and healthcare, simple access to technology, but also people's ability and willingness to use it are critical for enabling tools for evidence-based practice in healthcare and education settings. Trends in healthcare related to the transition from acute to chronic diseases affecting larger parts of the developed country population, increased coordination and professionalism of patients, the introduction of electronic patient files and increasing penetration of the Internet affect health information and communication.

Recent developments in traditional healthcare have been associated with the concept of intelligent and communicative patients [4]. Today, patients are educated people demanding a healthcare system that respects their rights and meets their needs. Patients are increasingly being considered in healthcare. All these developments require adapting conventional health information tools and developing new tools in response to patient demand and health information needs.

Many health information sources are freely available on the Internet, but little is known about the social and economic consequences. These processes emphasize that technologies that focus on patient communication and provide patient-tailored information are important for shared decision-making and for an open healthcare system where patients become partners in part or all of treatment.

Telemedicine/home monitoring solutions are also an attractive concept owing to their broad usability and possibilities for remote, personalized feedback. However, patient participation requires further developments in medical informatics, clinical specialization, epidemiology and health economics in collaboration with patients.

The future will show that eHealth and new business models that involve patients and healthcare on a social level can disrupt and change traditional healthcare [5]. The focus should be on engaging all stakeholders—patients and their representatives—in the research, definition, implementation and evaluation of such e-health activities and projects. Such activities and projects include the development of technology-assisted health information systems for the secure exchange of critical patient health information at the point of care for evidence-based medical decision-making and coordinated patient-centric care. A broad, complementary strategy to promote e-services and self-management as innovation carriers for healthcare should also consider information and communication technology capabilities for supporting health promotion and health literacy among stakeholders in healthcare. This will rethink healthcare and the role of stakeholders in a new interactive relationship, promoting citizen and patient empowerment. Such questions must be coordinated and balanced within the activities, planning and funding for eHealth.

3.1 Electronic health records (EHRs)

Electronic Health Records are tools developed to assist care providers in improving the quality, safety, efficiency and effectiveness of healthcare service delivery to patients and populations. The aim of EHRs is to make clinical records more transparent while avoiding quality attrition. Electronic health records must include the full life histories of a patient's health status and enable treatment decision-making by care providers who can tailor measures to patient and family concerns. EHRs also support patient-centered, evidenced-based health communication and collaboration among care team members when operated safely and securely. A robust healthcare delivery is possible with an optimal EHR system aiming at better health outcomes, better patient/provider experiences and lower healthcare costs. Communications regarding patient health data and best practices between clinical providers of primary care services for all their assigned patients and across a region are key to meaningful practice transformation [6]. In short, EHRs, designed to make clinical record keeping more transparent and to prevent healthcare quality erosion, are tools used by care providers to improve the quality, safety, efficiency and effectiveness of healthcare service delivery to patients and populations.

3.2 Clinical decision support systems

Clinical decision support systems (CDSS) support clinicians in providing evidence-based, patient-specific healthcare. CDSS uses two main data strands: By matching individual patient healthcare data with computerized clinical knowledge and by recommending evidence-based clinical practice guidelines to healthcare providers. Providing general information, decision support or access to specific disease management applications, CDSS are designed to enhance patient care quality and safety through advanced clinical information systems and care management support. Knowledge-based CDSS are computers that use a database of information together with a set of provable facts and heuristics to make decisions or give structured advice. Known CDSS examples include those that use signs and symptoms, history and physical examination to guide medical decisions.

Potential benefits for clinical decision support systems include the ability to provide detailed, comprehensive and therapy-related patient-specific information to the healthcare provider. Clinical decision support tools lead to an improved process of healthcare delivery. Knowledge embedded in clinical logic is applied systematically for improved healthcare cost-effectiveness, patient outcomes and patient satisfaction. Identification and resolution of key structural, process and care management issues are critical steps to integrating decision support into CDSS systems.

3.3 Telemedicine and remote monitoring

Telemedicine is among the most frequently mentioned medical applications of advanced telecommunications involving videoconferencing, store and forward technologies and real-time consumer monitoring. For remote monitoring people can collect and send vital signs to physicians working remotely. Several pediatric cardiology programs have begun telemedicine encounters in intensive care units and neonatal intensive care units across geographical boundaries. This may reduce costs, increase patient and staff satisfaction and improve outcomes. Telemedicine and remote monitoring are also developed. Together, augmented reality, telemedicine and remote patient monitoring through one infrastructure will improve workforce productivity and patient care. While current patient monitoring occurs in the walls of healthcare institutions, some successful trials using new-generation wearable sensors coupled with developments in information and communication technology allow remote monitoring of patient signs of health. Such monitoring makes the organization of clinical trials in other environments—like homes, schools and other locations—easier, faster and less expensive. Opportunities include technical detection and quantification of specific signals of ADHD, depression, fatigue, physical activity and other behavioral health conditions for automated, objective, real-time assessment.

All these technological efforts should aim at better understanding individual patients' emotional, cognitive or physical states and capacities for acquiring, processing or understanding knowledge. But it is also true that patient-family collaboration as well as research, philanthropic and healthcare industry collaboration can help us not only use new technologies but also mitigate the negative effects.

4. Big data and analytics in evidence-based healthcare

More recently, efforts to use big data and formal analytics in health and medicine are also being applied, as well as electronic records and decision support applications. Yet the health sciences are now joining in too—sometimes because they already handle data well. For example, clinical trials apply many principles and methods of formal analytics. Additionally, health-related big data has been analyzed across social science and economics, as well as biochemistry and genomic technologies have changed biomedical research by generating huge amounts of genetic and epigenetic data that often promise personalized therapy and drug discovery [7]. Many recent and ongoing works on formal analytics in evidence have been funded by digital health startups and apps, often just empty shells of ideas rather than real businesses that may all vanish, change or be taken over but which today are more than just hype that traditional health investors and healthcare conglomerates do not ignore, even when mostly unfunded by academic grants.

4.1 Definition and significance

Two associated forces convert otherwise well-meaning random and selective applications of information into the best national policy and method of practice. One is the ever-growing application of science that is becoming more applied to technology. The other one is the healthcare financing that creates new industrial forms of organizations bigger than ever before, targeting small sector services they need. Such demands involve additional costs, more punctuality, better professional self-discipline, and higher accountability through performance measurement. Together, they are making uncritical application of medical expertise a thing of the past in policy and practice. Such expertise is only permissible if all demands can be met—most of the time. The question will be academic soon enough—with or without us—except perhaps as medical sociology and an account of what might have been if conscious control had not been exercised in implementing a best-evidence method of care [8]. The definition is always the same—care according to procedures that have best-resisted assessment by scientific methods. But to be useful, its constantly changing assumptions must become reality in practice.

4.2 Applications in healthcare

One of the pioneers in the use of computers to aid health professionals in making decisions and solving problems was Dr. Douglas Perot Robertson. The diseases for which he designed consultative programs addressed some of the major health problems that many doctors encountered regularly. Today's computer-literate doctors are excited about computers. Daily, computer technology makes the impossible problems of yesterday look so easy. Such advancements have always presented new choices. They are developing more varied algorithms and strategies for their use. Because we know they are good for our patients' health, many of us are replacing low-technology ways. It is logical therefore to ask "What is the bottom line?"

Saying there is evidence that many high-technology ways of doing things are more effective than traditional low-technology ways is rather simplistic [9]. The problem is that benefits from high technology are generally greater, more certain and more predictable. This latter aspect of the discussion is why, in the end, technology will change healthcare. Our low-tech ways of diagnosing and treating the current patient population are problem-solving mechanisms. A conceptual breakthrough in terms of technology has been the finding in modern science that diseases arise from manipulable conditions [10, 11]. As they occur somewhat independently of the hereditary and environmental determinants of each patient, the benefits of diagnosis and management based on the successful manipulation of the conditions can be quite predictable. Thanks to scientific advances, today the diagnostic and therapeutic technologies required to manipulate most of these conditions are modern and highly sophisticated. Their utility potential is barely scratched.

5. Artificial intelligence (AI) and machine learning (ML) in transforming healthcare

A famous joke says that half of everything learned in medical school turns out to be false—but nobody knows which half. Evidence-based medicine is the foundation of good clinical practice—physicians, patients and payers all benefit from applying scientific knowledge to medical decision-making and patient care. What may be unexpected in the context of such improved just-in-time evidence delivery is the relatively low real-time adoption of this critical information by clinicians who are directly delivering the benefit to their patients. Up till now, electronic health records have mainly enabled the repeated characterization of the resistance of clinical practices toward periodic scientific revolutions [12, 13].

Newer technologies in artificial intelligence and machine learning may change this by offering fundamentally different ways of information delivery. Large-scale phenotypic data extraction from unstructured portions of the electronic health record permits near-real-time signal-noise evaluation of existing knowledge for the development of predictive algorithms to support evidence discovery [14]. Those same tools can also test and implement these new algorithms; models can help front-line clinicians apply knowledge more consistently and in the timely generation of new observational studies, pragmatic clinical trials and other primary data required to provide critical new evidence. The advent of machine learning allows this new world of real-time data to reach unprecedented levels of information for our clinical decision-makers. Applied to the right circumstances, artificial intelligence may 1 day help our customers with just-in-time care.

5.1 AI and ML: Introduction

AI/ML is increasingly used in healthcare settings, including diagnosis/treatment selection/monitoring of patient outcomes, billing, engagement and public health. AI/ML solutions can impact on care delivery/data flow by highlighting existing inequalities and biases. It is imperative that any health system transformation resulting from such new methods is guided by principles of improved net care delivery and a determination to develop methods of AI/ML oversight and accountability [15]. This chapter describes the current state and near-term outlook for AI/ML in healthcare and its application to the process of gathering and using evidence-based healthcare data.

Healthcare professionals increasingly use technological devices to interface with electronic health records and code and document patient encounters. As the overflow of clinical, administrative and research data becomes structured, AI and ML are having an impact. The term ML can refer to any combination of supervised, unsupervised and reinforcement methods used to train algorithms to make predictions, discover new characteristics or optimize responses. The example of AI driven by machine learning is one example of the emergence of health technology, which can be defined broadly as "the application of scientific knowledge for practical purposes." Particular health technology applications, powered by ML, generally fall under the umbrella term e-health, which refers to the provision of healthcare over the Internet, telecommunications and increasingly mobile apps.

5.2 Using cases in evidence-based healthcare

Let us consider the following case: a patient makes an appointment with their primary care physician after learning of a disturbing change in their symptoms. The primary care physician reports this new cancer progression to the oncologist, who adjusts the patient's chemotherapy plan for this progression. A revised chemotherapy plan is developed, the appointment is concluded and the patient returns home with little disruption to the day. That happened because monitoring data from a wearable health device alerted a primary care physician, who could attend to the issue at their scheduled appointment.

Such data-driven, real-time and patient-centered coordination of care across a variety of digital health technologies for patient outcomes does not represent what most patient-healthcare providers encounter today [16]. However, using cases such as the one above might yield considerable evidence to inform future models of evidence-based healthcare. In such evolving models of evidence-based healthcare, the priority is to systematically integrate broad and varied patient-centered data relevant to patient needs and outcomes to enable a more individualized healthcare approach. Participants consider the specific features of evidence-based healthcare models—convergence strategies, clinical, regulatory and reimbursement trends—that will define and enable patient-centered methodologies—and discuss the opportunities and challenges of next-generation healthcare. We generally accept that this model may produce some important outcomes. Not only does it have to search for and act upon signals predictive of poor patient outcomes, but such interventions are most effective when they can do so while maintaining a patient-centered quality of life. Such models address patient and physician concerns in a way that combines new therapies while remaining within pain, symptom and functionality limits set by each patient's needs and values.

6. Challenges and ethical issues in technology-enabled evidence-based healthcare

Challenges and ethical issues in technology-enabled evidence-based healthcare have changed healthcare access, delivery and outcomes at many levels. There are challenges and ethical questions, though. The first challenge is the possible digital health disparity, where technology is not universally available or is used differently depending on age, education and digital literacy. Hence, equity in access to and within technology-enabled interventions is needed to ensure the participation of the vulnerable population. It is thought that technology is being adopted most readily by young people but not by most existing health conditions.

Technologist-enabled evidence-based healthcare is rapidly evolving alongside new ethical challenges that require higher professional and ethical standards. The underlying research that interacts with health technology must be transparent, rigorous and unbiased [17, 18]. Patient access to information sources and the associated shared decision-making also need to be based on evidence rather than marketing or commercial perspectives. Health professionals should consider the positives and negatives in deciding how to personalize technology-enabled big data research embedded in evidence-based healthcare. Finally, in seeking this balance, health professionals and patients need to remember that digital health cannot replace the patient-practitioner relationship.

6.1 Privacy and security

All technologies approach privacy and security in terms of design and policy. The data must be sufficient for the system's purpose and actual use case, not more. Such questions must have a policy dimension and be overseen clearly by citizens who can hold designers, policymakers and operations accountable. Those covered by regulation include health plans, healthcare clearinghouses and some healthcare providers. Pioneering efforts are being developed to remove personally identifiable characteristics such as people with sensitive records [19, 20].

And data access is important too. Privacy/security issues must be managed so as not to restrict access to health data. Data stewardship is one facet of responsible health data access. All sorts of groups have data about us as people—from our doctors, hospitals and insurance companies to technology, data mining and marketing companies in other countries. Such entities decide on data that affects our everyday lives but lack clear accountability. The maxim "it is not your data unless you delete it" is a common refrain, but getting enough assurance for interested parties to take data beyond the bounds of individual liability is not always easy [21].

6.2 Bias and fairness

Bias and fairness are generally considered as necessary requirements for decision-making, particularly in healthcare. Automated processes have to be fair to the vulnerability of assignments without excluding or disadvantaging any particular group or being unfair in decision-making or representation. Moreover, principles of the Global Good Clinical (GGC) practice require that information relating to and based on individuals' personal data must be kept confidential and safe. This new opportunity is to frame bias and fairness at the development stage of AI, consequently ensuring GGC principles. These required conditions are not only ethical but legally binding requirements [22]. Secondly, make algorithms more transparent and understandable so that systems can communicate their accuracy, and thirdly, Demonstrable results, repeatability and predictability, safe inputs/secure outputs, easy-to-define human accountability, internal and external adaptation capacity, optimal performance. Conclusion: the big question is social pressure. Society should demand effective, equitable and ethical technologies; governments should regulate and promote ethical development. The principle of choosing is indispensable. These bias problems may result in denying opportunities or cutting costs for people most familiar with a hierarchical social group versus people less familiar with that group. A new explanation for the generalization of the fairness principle appears: treatment neutrality. A fairness principle is then applied because of similarities. This principle is also detailed in the measurement and allocation of losses due to automation. Finally, distributive justice considers the fairness principle. For health, multidisciplinary teams need multidimensional strategic, legal and quantitative stakeholders to enable accountable health innovation [23].

7. Future trends and innovations in technology and evidence-based healthcare

The future of evidence-based healthcare is intertwined with technology in three fundamental ways: a single set of scientific data may have many different uses and be analyzed for these uses; All healthcare decisions will become rapidly chaotic with many, large, complex data sources beyond the reach of most decision makers. And now, their related secondary challenges—namely, the developmental gap between explicitly instructive evidence summaries and the needs of decision-makers—are becoming more prominent in the digitally interconnected community of the future [24, 25]. This section discusses some of the medical and technological innovations that may disrupt evidence-based medicine practice in the future—combining existing data and clinical information, patient-centered decision support systems based on whole genome information and personalized mobile healthcare for the digital native.

The best evidence for a healthcare decision is evidence-based care. Its convenience—that is, to what extent is information available for use and support of an appropriate health outcome for a given patient or a given population. And transparency—how easily the decision can be explained to others. The fact that evidence-based care is about selecting rather than performing tasks makes it naturally granular. In practice, however, the generation and evaluation of the underlying clinical or scientific evidence for healthcare has been transforming the way decision-making occurs in healthcare practice. Using a strong body of medical evidence can increase safety in healthcare, reduce medical costs by standardizing procedures and improve outcomes.

7.1 Precision medicine

Such developments in the digital and data-driven worlds have enabled us to predict risk and pinpoint treatments that are likely to work for whom. This is called precision medicine in healthcare. Some of the most promising new developments in diagnostic testing are improved microarrays or in-silico pathology. Ultra-sensitive tests using biomarkers to detect cancer or other diseases early or to detect disease recurrence after treatment, have been demonstrated outside the laboratory context. Still others say progress toward practical diagnostic tests is lagging behind fundamental advances in our knowledge of the disease. The authors also point out how these diagnostic tests may affect cancer treatment, possible overdiagnosis and overtreatment [26].

The many promising new treatments for rare diseases include gene replacement therapy, gene editing, stem cell therapy and mobilizing the latent disease-fighting power of the human microbiome. Potential ethical questions regarding progress in therapies targeting rare genetic diseases include who should receive the limited research funding, how to address gaps in access to high-cost, high-tech medicine or public health initiatives and what our obligations are regarding returning benefits to populations participating in the research. This incredible pace of advance in precision medicine leaves audiences at big expos thinking that the first generation of personalized or precision medicine is almost here. Still, questions remain and challenges persist including regulatory issues surrounding personalized/precision medicine, mechanisms for data sharing/storage and barriers to affordability.

7.2 Internet of Things (IoT)

The heterogeneity of illness behaviors, health determinants, lifestyles and willingness and ability to use technology may limit the application of various products and services to specific populations' health. Some groups may find health applications especially effective: For example, older adults who report feeling fatigued or disabled. Individuals have one to three chronic conditions. And those who fit certain behavioral profiles, such as needing to avoid routine physical visits. Yet, complexity, distrust, privacy issues related to data security and misuse of data, cost and subject expertise, and digital literacy to use tools effectively are becoming increasingly challenging for the poorest and most vulnerable in the world [27].

Despite these problems, devices and user interfaces could increasingly be adapted to overcome low health literacy. New technologies/care models may be the central focus of personalized/predictive/preventive/participatory medicine. By 2025, the global wearable medical devices market size is estimated to be around USD 53.73 billion in 2025 and rise to around USD 427.05 billion by 2034 at a compound annual growth rate (CAGR) of 25.90% from 2025 to 2034 [28]. Identities could be identified using shorthand or scanned with a smartphone. In addition to partners and patients, individuals and patient groups armed with smart devices may become increasingly powerful and expect more control over health data or a better understanding of genetic data. Highly modified public data is distributed among value and market share. So, looking at how new technologies might improve efficiency, break monopolies and increase accessibility might, therefore, potentially help the technology and commercial landscape work for patients.

8. Conclusion

Evidence-based healthcare applies the best evidence from research and health practice to health decisions for individuals, healthcare systems and healthcare policymakers. This helps optimize patient outcomes and healthcare costs. Still, healthcare practices have not shifted to an evidence-based approach quickly or completely. Technological promises may enable evidence-based healthcare. The chapter identifies the many ways that technology supports evidence-based healthcare, provides examples of new tools/approaches and challenges to overcome to ensure ongoing innovation, testing and implementation. For instance, evaluation deployment using decision support tools, digital data exchange interconnectivity, artificial intelligence applications, technological advances in population health research and system architecture are direct examples of the successful results of these investments.

Transformation of the economic efficiency and effectiveness of some healthcare requires a new technological advance. But a significant proportion depends on obtaining the best use of available evidence. Politicians have tried to force evidence-based coverage, payment and health service quality oversight. However, compliance with the various health information technology implementation stipulations was low, although recognition that even the best evidence may be obsolete in 5 years was expressed.

8.1 Key points

This chapter asks whether the assumed evidence-based changes are really happening because of a wave of techno-social innovations in relation to big data, which are described as transformative for healthcare use. It focuses on three empirical examples cited by other authors that might be representative of big data just starting to change healthcare. The three are thus framed within the normative dimensions of EBHC in terms of the three signifying clusters of value tensions regarding choices regarding individual freedoms versus collective good or benefits and harms versus long- and short-term outcomes. The Triple Helix of data, discussions and decision-making can, therefore, be viewed as a framework that can enhance the valuation choices of actors in this space. Observations regarding big data in healthcare are based on foundational theory and are recognized as determinants of patient and societal health and costs across different health contexts. In taking into account a Socio-Technical Perspective this chapter raises a question mark of purported evidence-based health care changes resulting from the cluster of related techno-social innovations. Information and communication technology is often promoted as a driver of technological innovation in society—including in healthcare. Big data in healthcare is offered as transformative as large health-related datasets become more common and easier to analyze. As normative dimensions of EBHC, they denote different clusters of value tensions about choices with respect to individual freedoms and collective good choices, benefits/ harms and long- and short-term outcomes. Thus, the Triple Helix of data, discussions and decision-making may be described as a framework that can enrich the valuation choices of actors in this space. Observations regarding big data in healthcare may be informed by foundational theory and recognized as determinants of patient and societal health and costs in various health contexts.

8.2 Implications for the future of healthcare

What does the future hold for healthcare? We know technology will affect all areas of healthcare. Already, it is transforming the medical office, the hospital and the research lab. Now, the physician has the most complete medical record ever created in the medical office. That makes obtaining references to literature as current as the previous day's publications somewhat intimidating for the patient and physician. Most routine laboratory testing that is low in functionality will be outsourced to automated services. Most diagnoses are entered and screened by computerization. But the most critical tool of the doctor—the judgment and advice based on experience—will always be a trait peculiar to humans. And in hospitals, technology offers more and more advanced care for the sick and injured, with a focus on cellular-level interventions. Because specialized hospitals increasingly provide surgical and acute care functions to adults, general hospitals will probably concentrate more heavily on pre- and post-hospital care services such as rehabilitation, mental health services and geriatrics.

A need exists in the concurrent domain of hospital nursing to foster creativity in bedside care—an enormous shift from the technical procedures that historically defined the discipline. Technological progress at the bedside appears to have plateaued, as the fully artificial patient has not yet been invented. The present system of research and testing is perhaps stricter than in any other field because of the direct and profound impact of financial outlays. Currently, there exists an almost universal cynicism about how medical research funding should be spent to meet the pressing social needs [29]. That discomfort is philosophical rather than practical, for the basic problem of our time is how to make successive generations of investments in the hardware and software systems of technology systematically integrated for true interoperability besides the data they handle. Not enough people understand what we are trying to achieve. Among competing priorities, divergence in visions of what can be done to improve the effectiveness and efficiency of healthcare forces divergent factions to take different courses. The real losers here will undoubtedly be the patients themselves, who will probably suffer the most from these badly coordinated efforts [30].

Author details

Elisabeta Shehu Kafia
Albanian University, Tirana, Albania

*Address all correspondence to: elisabetakafia@yahoo.co.uk

References

[1] Erku D, Khatri R, Endalamaw A, Wolka E, Nigatu F, Zewdie A, et al. Digital health interventions to improve access to and quality of primary health care services: A scoping review. International Journal of Environmental Research and Public Health. 2023;**20**(19):6854. Published 2023 Sep 28. DOI: 10.3390/ijerph20196854

[2] Mumtaz H, Riaz MH, Wajid H, et al. Current challenges and potential solutions to the use of digital health technologies in evidence generation: A narrative review. Frontiers in Digital Health. 2023;**5**:1203945. Published 2023 Sep 28. DOI: 10.3389/fdgth.2023.1203945

[3] Dwivedi Y, Kshetri N, Hughes L, Rana N, Baabdullah A, Kar A, et al. Exploring the darkverse: A multi-perspective analysis of the negative societal impacts of the metaverse. Information Systems Frontiers. 2023;**25**:2071-2114

[4] Garin N, Sole N, Lucas B, Matas L, Moras D, Rodrigo-Troyano A, et al. Drug related problems in clinical practice: A cross-sectional study on their prevalence, risk factors and associated pharmaceutical interventions. Scientific Reports. 2021;**11**:883, 1-11. DOI: 10.1038/s41598-020-80560-2

[5] Jabarulla MY, Lee H-N. A blockchain and artificial intelligence-based, patient-centric healthcare system for combating the COVID-19 pandemic: Opportunities and applications. Healthcare. 2021;**9**:1019. DOI: 10.3390/healthcare9081019

[6] Rani S, Kataria A, Kumar S, Tiwari P. Federated learning for secure IoMT-applications in smart healthcare systems: A comprehensive review. Knowledge-Based Systems. 2023;**274**:110658. DOI: 10.1016/j.knosys.2023.110658

[7] Iyanna S, Kaur P, Ractham P, Talwar S, Islam AKM. Digital transformation of healthcare sector. What is impeding adoption and continued usage of technology-driven innovations by end-users? Journal of Business Research. 2022;**153**:150-161. DOI: 10.1016/j.jbusres.2022.08.007

[8] Kraus S, Schiavone F, Pluzhnikova A, Invernizzi A. Digital transformation in healthcare: Analyzing the current state-of-research. Journal of Business Research. 2020;**123**:557-567. DOI: 10.1016/j.jbusres.2020.10.030

[9] Cremin CJ, Dash S, Huang X. Big data: Historic advances and emerging trends in biomedical research. Current Research in Biotechnology. 2022;**4**:138-151. DOI: 10.1016/j.crbiot.2022.02.004

[10] Teede HJ, Tay CT, Laven JJ, Dokras A, Moran LJ, Piltonen TT, et al. Recommendations from the 2023 international evidence-based guideline for the assessment and management of polycystic ovary syndrome. European Journal of Endocrinology. 2023;**189**(2):G43-G64. Available from: https://oup.com

[11] Susskind R, Susskind D. The future of the professions. Proceedings of the American Philosophical Society. 2018;**162**(2). Available from: https://www.amphilsoc.org/sites/default/files/2018-11/attachments/Susskind%20and%20Susskind.pdf

[12] Jaeger L, Dacorogna M. Biology from 1953 to 2023: Major breakthroughs and their ethical issues: How biology became

the centre of science and today also lies at the centre of ethical concerns. In: Where Is Science Leading Us? And What Can We Do to Steer It? Springer Nature Switzerland: Cham; 2024. pp. 147-174. [HTML]

[13] Montero DA, Vidal RM, Velasco J, Carreño LJ, Torres JP, Benachi OMA, et al. Two centuries of vaccination: Historical and conceptual approach and future perspectives. Frontiers in Public Health. 2024;**11**:1326154. Available from: https://frontiersin.org

[14] Wei WQ, Denny JC. Extracting research-quality phenotypes from electronic health records to support precision medicine. Genome Medicine. 2015;**7**(1):41. DOI: 10.1186/s13073-015-0166-y

[15] Nersessian NJ. Interdisciplinarity in the Making: Models and Methods in Frontier Science. Cambridge, Massachusetts: The MIT Press; 2022

[16] Brands MR, Gouw SC, Beestrum M, Cronin RM, Fijnvandraat K, Badawy SM. Patient-centered digital health records and their effects on health outcomes: Systematic review. Journal of Medical Internet Research. 2022;**24**(12):e43086. DOI: 10.2196/43086

[17] Wang C, Liu S, Yang H, Guo J, Wu Y, Liu J. Ethical considerations of using ChatGpt in health care. Journal of Medical Internet Research. 2023;**25**:e48009. DOI: 10.2196/48009

[18] Garcia M, Garcia P, Maaliw R III, Lagrazon P, Arif Y, Ofosu-Ampong K, et al. Technoethical considerations for advancing health literacy and medical practice: A posthumanist framework in the age of healthcare 5.0. 2024. DOI: 10.4018/979-8-3693-1214-8.ch001

[19] Haleem A, Javaid M, Singh RP, Suman R. Medical 4.0 technologies for healthcare: Features, capabilities, and applications. Internet of Things and Cyber-Physical Systems. 2022;**2**:12-30. Available from: https://sciencedirect.com

[20] Badnjevic A. Evidence-based maintenance of medical devices: Current shortage and pathway towards solution. Technology and Health Care. 2023;**31**:293-305. DOI: 10.3233/THC-229005

[21] Wager KA, Lee FW, Glaser JP. Health Care Information Systems. 5th ed. Wiley; 2021. Available from: https://www.perlego.com/book/3118785/health-care-information-systems-a-practical-approach-for-health-care-management-pdf

[22] Filip R, Gheorghita Puscaselu R, Anchidin-Norocel L, Dimian M, Savage WK. Global challenges to public health care systems during the COVID-19 pandemic: A review of pandemic measures and problems. Journal of Personalized Medicine. 2022;**12**(8):1295. Available from: https://mdpi.com

[23] McIntosh T, Susnjak T, Liu T, Xu D, Watters P, Liu D, et al. Ransomware reloaded: Re-examining its trend, research and mitigation in the era of data exfiltration. ACM Computing Surveys. 2024;**57**(1):1-40. Available from: https://acm.org

[24] Junaid SB, Imam AA, Balogun AO, De Silva LC, Surakat YA, Kumar G, et al. Recent advancements in emerging technologies for healthcare management systems: A survey. Healthcare (Basel, Switzerland). 2022;**10**(10):1940. DOI: 10.3390/healthcare10101940

[25] Almujadidi B, Adams A, Alquaiz A, Van Gurp G, Schuster T, Andermann A. Exploring social determinants of health in a Saudi Arabian primary health care setting: The need for a multidisciplinary

approach. International Journal for Equity in Health. 2022;**21**(1):24. Available from: https://springer.com

[26] Letterie G. Three ways of knowing: The integration of clinical expertise, evidence-based medicine, and artificial intelligence in assisted reproductive technologies. Journal of Assisted Reproduction and Genetics. 2021;**38**(7):1617-1625. DOI: 10.1007/s10815-021-02159-4

[27] Stein DJ, Shoptaw SJ, Vigo DV, Lund C, Cuijpers P, Bantjes J, et al. Psychiatric diagnosis and treatment in the 21st century: Paradigm shifts versus incremental integration. World Psychiatry. 2022;**21**(3):393-414. Available from: https://wiley.com

[28] Wearable Medical Devices Market Size, Share, and Trends 2025 to 2034. Available from: https://www.precedenceresearch.com/wearable-medical-device-market

[29] Lim G, Kam AJY. Chinese Investment in Malaysia: (De)industrialization amidst greater financial and trade connectivity. The European Journal of Development Research; Palgrave Macmillan; European Association of Development Research and Training Institutes (EADI). 2024;**36**(3):571-600

[30] Igwama GT, Olaboye JA, Maha CC, Ajegbile MD, Abdul S. Integrating electronic health records systems across borders: Technical challenges and policy solutions. International Medical Science Research Journal. 2024;**4**(7):788-796

Chapter 5

Development of a Framework for the Integrated Management of Falls within the Residential Care Home Setting for Older Persons in Malta: An Evidence-Based Approach

Matthew Cini, Ingrid Flores and Patricia Vella Bonanno

Abstract

Falls are a major concern for older persons living in residential care home settings, often leading to significant injuries, and affecting their quality of life. Falls management is part of the governance framework at all levels of care in a healthcare system: macro, meso and micro levels. Residential care homes should implement a holistic and comprehensive falls management system to reduce the rate of falls and prevent fall-related injuries. This study aimed to develop a falls management framework for older persons living in the Maltese residential care home setting, which is currently lacking. A critically appraised topic (CAT) of the literature was conducted to build a conceptual falls management framework. The conceptual framework was evaluated by comparison with different international falls management frameworks. Evidence from stakeholders at different levels (regulators, care home managers, healthcare professionals and residents) was collected. Participants prioritised the elements, categories and components represented in the conceptual model. The participants older persons had a different perspective compared to the other stakeholders, when prioritising the elements. The results were used to develop an evidence-based falls management framework for Malta.

Keywords: evidence-based, framework, falls management, stakeholders, residential care homes, system levels, older person, regulation, organisational level, operational level, healthcare professionals, healthcare systems

1. Introduction

The World Health Organisation (WHO) defined a fall as "an event which results in a person coming to rest inadvertently on the ground or floor or other lower level" [1]. Falls are a common symptom of ageing, and the risk increases as a person ages [2, 3]. Falls are particularly more prevalent in a residential care home setting, compared to community-dwelling older persons [3, 4]. Falls are associated with negative repercussions, including increased morbidity, fracture, head injuries, bleeding, disability, residential care home admissions and death [1, 5–7]. Moreover, a fall can affect the mental well-being of an older person either due to fear of sustaining another fall leading to a sedentary lifestyle, or depressive symptoms, which are associated with an increased disability brought about by a fall [6]. The high prevalence of falls and their negative repercussions cause a huge burden on the older person and the healthcare system [1, 8] and falls must be managed. An effective falls management system can prevent fall-associated complications and reduce the risk of future falls [9]. Montero-Odasso et al. supported this and added that falls management could also help with improving the well-being and general health of older persons worldwide [10].

1.1 The residential care home system for older persons

A systems approach is critical to manage adverse events, including falls, and to improving patient safety and quality care [10, 11]. The system is a highly complex interaction between system levels, resources and organisations, all networking together to deliver good quality care [12, 13].

The World Health Organisation (WHO) defined the healthcare system "as comprising all the organisations, institutions and resources that are devoted to producing health actions" [14]. The residential care home system could be considered as a subsystem of the healthcare system, which relates to it through a level of integration [15]. The main aim of the residential care home is to promote quality of life and maintain dignity [16]. The residential care home system is indefinite and ongoing, providing good quality care to older persons who were not able to live independently in the community. This system of care offers a more specialised level of care, which is not feasible in the community. The residential care home is designed specifically to facilitate older persons to conduct activities of daily living. Moreover, specialised services are provided according to the older person's care plan, including services by allied health professionals and specialised nursing [16].

A residential care home system involves a broad range of stakeholders and service providers, each with distinct roles and responsibilities to ensure quality service for older persons [17]. The system's functionality depends on the interactions between various levels, with its emergence relying on exchanged among these levels. These interconnected levels from an integrated system, each relying on the others [12, 18]. Implementing a falls management system in residential care homes requires input and contribution from stakeholders across all levels to ensure safety, quality of care and quality improvement [19].

The residential care home system is based on three levels: macro, meso and micro [20]. These three levels determine quality and safety [21]. **Figure 1** is an adaptation of the model presented by Ciasullo et al. [22] which represents the system levels of a residential care home system.

At the macro level, regulation is integral, setting limits on what is acceptable or lawful [23]. Regulation aims to protect the public's interest to ensure safety, fairness and standards of quality and performance [24]. This is done in parallel to holding the service provider accountable, which strongly influences how organisations approach improvement [25].

The meso level involves managerial staff responsible for running residential care homes. Management acts as an intermediary, connecting the macro and micro levels to collaborate and provide value, including knowledge, expertise, and resources. This fulfils the service user's expectations and particular needs [12]. Meso-level actors ensure a system which gathers clinical information, allowing for the monitoring of various

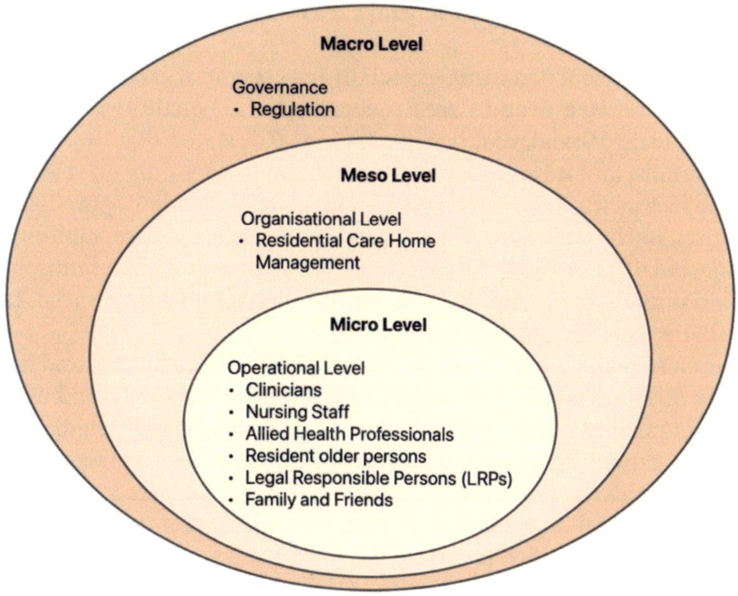

Figure 1.
Concentric circle model representing the residential care home system adapted from Ciasullo et al. [22].

components within the organisation. This compiled data presents the performance of the residential care home, which reflects on the general healthcare system [8].

The micro level represents the staff at the operational level, service users, and relatives or legal representatives. At this level, a dyad relationship is present between the healthcare provider and the service user, working together to manage and treat physical and mental well-being [23].

Shared knowledge guides all levels to develop individualised strategies to minimise fall rates [23]. Quality improvement depends on the combination of work and harmony of all three levels [25]. Finally, responsibility and provision of good quality care are shared across all system levels [23].

1.2 The residential care home setting for older persons in Malta

In Malta, the operational entity responsible for services for older persons, the Active Ageing and Community Care (AACC) is under the responsibility of the Ministry for Health and Active Ageing [26]. At the time of completion of this study, AACC is responsible for 26 residential care homes: six are government homes, two are church homes, and the rest are private. Residents living in the church and private homes occupy beds under a Private Public Partnership (PPP) scheme. This partnership allows the home contractor to run the residential care home whilst the government pays for the bed occupancy and the service provided to the resident older person [27]. These residential care homes benefit from several services offered by AACC, including services of allied health professionals, specialised nursing services (tissue viability nurse, specialised continence nurse and dementia practice nurse) and psychotherapy [28]. All residential care homes in Malta are regulated by the Older Person Standards Authority (OPSA), which is within the Ministry for Health and Active Ageing. The OPSA strives to include the service users and providers to be actively involved in developing and enhancing standards [29].

1.3 Management of falls in the residential care home system for older persons

Falls are multifactorial in nature, especially in residential care homes [19]. The National Institute for Health and Care Excellence (NICE) quality standards, 'Falls in Older People - Quality Standards', last updated in 2017, stated that there are up to 400 risk factors for falls, and it is rare for an older person to have only one risk factor [30]. Common risk factors for falls are categorised into social and demographic factors, medical factors, medication side effects or polypharmacy, balance, mobility, sensory and neuromuscular factors [31]. NICE stated that as part of their minimum standards for falls, the risk assessment and the interventions must be multifactorial, targeting the older persons' specific needs [30].

Older persons are not a homogenous group [32]. They are diverse and heterogeneous, with different physical capabilities, functional capacities, and needs [33]. Moreover, older persons can present with varying levels of frailty, medications, and risk factors. Providing one standard level of care to all older persons, promotes the false idea that older persons are all the same. A person-centred approach with a specific care plan is vital. Seppala and Van Der Velde [31] emphasised the importance of fall risk stratification, which is carried out on admission to a residential care home and on a routine basis as standard practice [31]. The authors acknowledged that this could be challenging when considering the substantial number of risk factors which need to be considered and can be time-consuming for the staff. The fall stratification algorithm should consider injuries due to past falls, frequency of falls, frailty, ability to stand up from a fall and level of consciousness [31]. These recommendations were supported by Montero-Odasso et al. [10], who, in their 'World Guidelines for Falls Management', recommended risk stratification to assign risk and added the importance of linking risk stratification to a multifactorial intervention.

Panneman et al. [8] and Jia et al. [34] encourage policymakers and service providers to work towards a better falls management system. Implementing a falls management framework is cost-effective, making it cheaper to carry out fall prevention training (balance and strength training) than to treat fall-related injuries such as fractures and head injuries [8, 34, 35].

The setting of international frameworks [10, 36–38] involved a collaborative approach in the development of their falls management frameworks. The collaborative approach included stakeholders from different residential care home system levels: macro, meso and micro. This aligns with Stavropoulou et al. [39], who emphasised that the development of any document in any setting should gain perspective and input from all stakeholders involved [39]. Finally, since a person-centred approach is considered standard practice, the older person, at the micro level should also be included in the development of a falls management framework [31].

1.4 Rationale and aim of this study

Malta does not have a comprehensive national framework for falls management across the different levels of the residential care home system. The management of falls in the local scenario mainly entails healthcare professionals at the operational level working together conducting a multifactorial risk assessment and post-fall management. The care home managers at the organisational level gather data, which is analysed and shared with OPSA and AACC, allowing the formulation of fall rate trends. Such as framework could guide stakeholders to manage falls more effectively and systematically.

Evidence-based practice is the standard across healthcare providers, organisations, and regulatory bodies [40]. It seeks to ensure and improve care quality, reduce adverse events and errors [41].

The aim of this study was to develop a framework for falls management in Malta, using an evidence-based approach.

2. Adopting an evidence-based approach for the development of falls management framework for Malta

2.1 Using the evidence-based model by Barends and Rousseau to design the study

The evidence-based management model by Barends and Rousseau [42] emphasises the collection of evidence from different sources of evidence including the literature, stakeholders, experts in the field and organisational data. The model for evidence-based management by Barends and Rousseau [42] adopts the approach of asking a question, acquiring the evidence from different sources, appraising this evidence, aggregating it together, applying it to practice and assessing it after its use [42]. The collection of evidence from players from different levels of the system (refer to **Figure 1**) ensures that the development of such a framework is grounded in evidence-based practice including stakeholder insights to enhance its effectiveness and relevance [42]. As presented in **Figure 2**, the model by Barends and Roussau [42] was adapted to collect and use evidence for the formation of falls management framework for Malta.

Professional expertise was collected from practitioners through focus groups with healthcare professionals working in residential care homes. Stakeholder values and concerns were collected via semi-structured interviews with older persons from residential care homes and a regulatory professional who was nominated by OPSA. Organisational internal data was obtained through semi-structured interviews with managers from residential care homes. The collected evidence was appraised, aggregated, and triangulated to enhance its effectiveness.

2.2 Using evidence from the literature to compile a conceptual falls management framework

Scientific literature was consulted using a critically appraised topic (CAT) review [43]. A critically appraised topic (CAT) is a type of literature review which summarises and compiles the best evidence available in a standardised manner. It is a practical, effective, and efficient approach that integrates clinical research into clinical practice, ensuring systematicity and reducing biases [44]. The CAT for this study was carried out to set a conceptual framework for falls management within the residential care home setting.

The literature identified five main elements for the conceptual framework: post-fall management, preventative, predictive, regulatory-level involvement, and organisational-level involvement. Post-fall management involves the actions taken after a resident older person sustains a fall. The preventative element encompasses implementing necessary actions to prevent falls as much as possible. The predictive element represents all components required to anticipate falls. The organisational and regulatory level elements represent the involvement of the residential care home manager and regulation, respectively. Categories were identified for the

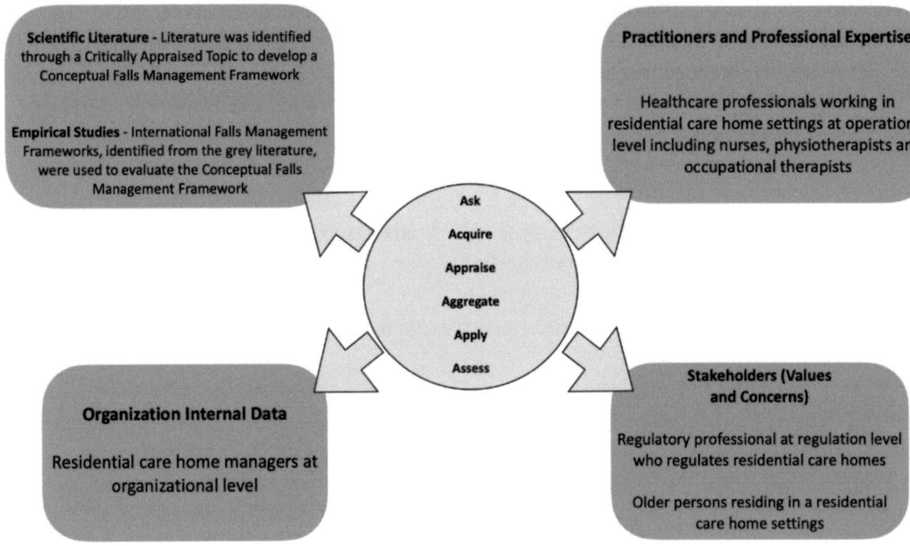

Figure 2.
Collection of evidence using the sources of evidence and the process for evaluation of the evidence as applied to this study, adapted from the model by Barends and Rousseau [42].

predictive element: multifactorial risk assessment, fall risk stratification and management. Categories were also identified for the post-fall management element: Procedural and participatory. Each element and category had respective components.

Eleven frameworks/guidelines for falls management were identified from the grey literature (**Table 1**). These were published by respected healthcare systems around the globe.

The elements, categories and components identified for each of these frameworks were tabulated and used to evaluate the conceptual framework. Each component was checked, and a percentage value was assigned, representing how much the particular component was included in the identified frameworks. Some changes were implemented to the conceptual framework. The Gait Speed Assessment Tool was only included in three frameworks as part of the assessment: “Preventing Falls and Harm from Falls in Older People” [52], “Preventing Falls and Reducing Injury from Falls” [37] and Reducing Falls and Injuries from Falls—Getting Started Kit [47]. Montero-Odasso et al. [10], Kyrdalen et al. [53], and Beck Jepsen et al. [54] stated that gait speed is a good predictor of falls in older persons. Moreover, the authors emphasise the importance of having this predictive tool as part of the multifactorial risk assessment and assessed regularly. The authors [54] also graded gait speed assessment tool as a 1A on the “grading of Recommendations, Assessment and Evaluation”, marking it as a strong recommendation. Therefore, this predictive, validated tool was kept in the conceptual falls management framework.

On the other hand, the frailty assessment tool was not included in any of the 11 frameworks from the grey literature. Thus, the component was excluded from the framework. The final conceptual falls management framework that was developed through the literature and evaluated through the models from the grey literature is presented in **Figure 3**.

Title	Entity/department	Nationality	Year
Falls: Standardised Care Process [45]	Victoria State Government: Department of Health and Human Services	Australia	2022
Procedure for the Prevention and Management of Adult Inpatients Falling in Hospital Settings [46]	National Health Service (NHS)	United Kingdom	2021 (reviewed)
Reducing Falls and Injuries from Falls – Getting Started Toolkit [47]	The Canadian Patient Safety Institute	Canada	2019
Post Fall Multidisciplinary Management Guidelines for Western Australian Health Care Settings [48]	Department of Health Government of Western Australia	Australia	2018
Service User Falls: A Practical Guide for Review [36]	Health Service Executive	Ireland	2018
Preventing Falls and Reducing Injury form Falls (4th Edition) [37]	International Affairs and Best Practice Guidelines (iaBPG)	Canada	2017
Falls Prevention Toolkit: Strategies for Streamlined Communication, Interdisciplinary Scope, and Patient and Family Engagement [38]	Missouri Hospital Association	United States	2014
Falls in Older People: Assessing Risk and Prevention [49]	The National Institute for Health and Care Excellence (NICE)	United Kingdom	2013
Preventing Falls in Hospitals: A Toolkit for Improving Quality of Care [50]	Agency for Healthcare Research and Quality	United States	2013
Falls and Related Injuries in Residential Care: A Framework and Toolkit for Prevention [51]	Centre of Excellence on Mobility, Fall Prevention and Injury in Ageing	Canada	2010
Preventing Falls and Harm from Falls in Older People [52]	Australian Commission on Safety and Quality in Healthcare	Australia	2009

Table 1.
Falls Management Frameworks and Guidelines.

2.3 Acquiring and appraising evidence from the different sources within the local setting

Information and prioritisation of the elements, categories, and components of the conceptual framework by different players (stakeholders, professionals and organisational managers) as shown in **Figure 2**, was conducted through mapping, using the Story Mapping Prioritisation Method by Patton and Economy [55]. This prioritisation aimed to fulfil two objectives: firstly, to identify which elements, categories, and components the players consider crucial for an effective falls management framework; and secondly, to prioritise them in order of their relative importance, from most to least relevant.

Two residential care homes were chosen, one from the private sector and one from the public sector. A set of inclusion and exclusion criteria were established, and participants were recruited by intermediaries using purposive sampling. This

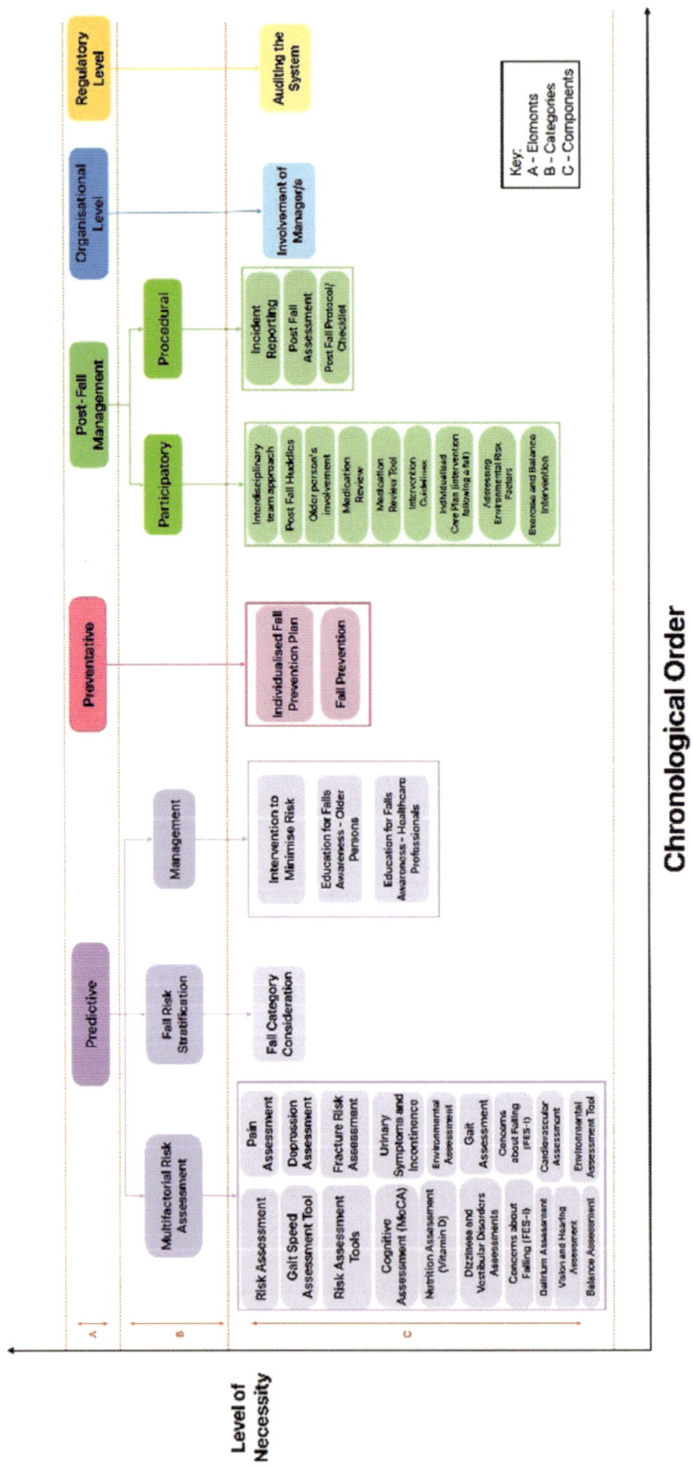

Figure 3.
Conceptual falls management framework.

sampling method was chosen to gather data from experts in the field who are part of the residential care home system.

Data collection commenced once permission was granted by the Faculty Research Ethics Committee for the Department of Social Wellbeing at the University of Malta. The description of the levels, participants and data collection method adopted for the respective participants is summarised in **Table 2**.

The prioritisations of the elements, categories, and components by each of the players were plotted onto mapping frameworks for better representation. All interviews and focus group meetings were transcribed for analysis. Reflexive thematic analysis was used to identify, analyse, and report themes from the gathered qualitative data relating to the stakeholders' perspective and expertise regarding the falls management framework in a residential care home setting. The stages of Braun and Clarke [56] were followed for thematic analysis. The frameworks as prioritised by different stakeholders were drawn and represented.

3. Aggregation of the evidence from the different sources

The evidence from the different players about the elements of the conceptual falls management framework (**Figure 2**) was aggregated to formulate a falls management framework for Malta.

3.1 Predictive element

The regulatory professional (RP), the managers and the healthcare professionals at the operational level all agreed and considered predictive as the most important element in falls management. The participant older persons placed this element as their second priority for falls management. The regulatory professional and organisational-level stakeholders explained that proper prediction of falls is the most effective way to prevent falls and fall-related injuries. Furthermore, predicting that a person has a high risk of falls can allow the healthcare team to modify the residential care home environment to prevent falls as much as possible. The players explained that it is their duty to predict adverse events before they occur. Predictive assessments should be carried out on admission, as routine and whenever indicated.

FG 1 Physiotherapist: *I think that's [carrying out a predictive assessment] the first step during admission, to determine if they have a higher risk to fall. I think the treatment should be based on the risk of the residents [older persons]. We can know what the resident [older person] needs from the risk assessment.*

The predictive element had three categories: (i) multifactorial risk assessment, (ii) fall risk stratification and (iii) management. The organisational and regulatory level stakeholders agreed by ranking the multifactorial risk assessment as the most important category in the predictive element. This was followed by fall risk stratification and then management. The RP described the first category as the definition of the element (predictive), meaning that a multifactorial risk assessment needs to be carried out to predict falls. The participant also added that falls are rarely caused by a single risk factor. Thus, having a multifactorial risk assessment is critical to predicting falls successfully.

M1: *...we have to assess for the risk so that we provide a specific, individualised plan, or programme... specific for the older persons. So we have to start with a robust assessment. And then... we would determine the risk [fall risk stratification], and assign the risk to each person.*

Stakeholder group (level)	Participants	Pseudonym	Inclusion criteria	Exclusion criteria	Data collection method
Regulatory level (macro)	• 1 regulatory professional from OPSA	RP	• Employed for a minimum of 1 year	• Newly appointed employees	Semi-structured interviews
Organisational level (meso)	• 1 manager of a private residential care home • 1 manager of a public residential care home	M1 & M2	• Employed for a minimum of 1 year	• Newly appointed employees • Employees on rotation	Semi-structured interviews
Operational level (micro)	• 1 focus group: healthcare professional at a private residential care home • 1 focus group: healthcare professional at a public residential care home	FG 1 & FG 2	• Employed for a minimum of 1 year	• Newly appointed employees • Employees on rotation	Focus Groups
Older person – the main stakeholder (micro)	• 2 participant older persons from a private residential care home • 2 participant older persons from a public residential care home	POP 1, POP 2, POP 3, & POP 4	• ≥60 years • Cognitively intact • Sustained a fall or recurrent fallers • Living in a residential care home for ≥6 months	• Cognitively impaired • Under a respite care plan	Semi-structured interviews

Table 2.
Participant demographic.

The healthcare professionals at operational level had a similar ranking, however, they considered fall risk stratification as important as a multifactorial risk assessment. The focus group participants discussed that the multifactorial risk assessment results should determine each older person-resident's risk stratification. The participants stated that every resident older person has a risk of falling, some more than others. However, identifying a person with a high risk of falls will allow the operational and organisational level to make the necessary changes to provide more supervision and equipment, and allocate them in a safe environment. Both categories form part of assessing the risk of falls; thus, both deserve the same rank.

FG 2 Physiotherapist: *All residents [older persons] should have an exercise programme, specific to them of course. They [older persons] should be categorised into different levels [high, medium and low risk]. So, we can provide more care.*

FG 2 Nurse: *We provide more supervision to those who have a higher risk of falls. Some of them [older persons], we keep them close to us, near the nursing station, so we can keep an eye on them.*

The participant older persons had a different perspective. They agreed that the multifactorial risk assessment category should be ranked in the first place and the management category in the second and final rank. However, they had mixed feelings about fall risk stratification. The majority of participant older persons did not understand the meaning of this category. One of the participants emphasised that everyone deserves a falls management program, regardless of the risk. Thus, the participant did not find stratification relevant to the falls management framework.

POP 1: *...but is not everyone entitled to care? So if he [name of roommate] falls more than me, and I only fall once, should not they [healthcare professionals] still come to review me? Everyone has a risk of falls. There's no need to categorise it...*

3.2 Preventative element

The participant older persons ranked the preventative element as their priority and related it to their negative past experiences associated with falls, fall-related injuries and increased dependence on others. Moreover, some participant older persons remarked that falls can be a reason for a residential care home admission, highlighting the importance of falls prevention. They emphasised the importance of not having to experience falls again and insisted that "*... prevention is better than cure*" (POP 1).

POP 2: *I always did everything myself. I took care of my mother and father. I did everything. After the fall, I ended waiting for them [the carers] to come to wash me. It's humiliating.*

The other stakeholders unanimously ranked the preventative element as their second priority. They considered that not all falls can be prevented, and all healthcare providers should ensure that everything is done to prevent falls as much as possible. They also emphasised that a fall prevention plan should be based on the findings of the multifactorial risk assessment to make it individualised, which overlaps with the predictive element.

RP: *...not all falls can be prevented. ... but it is our duty to make our absolute best to prevent falls as much as possible.*

FG 1 Occupational Therapist: *...from what we find in the [multifactorial risk] assessment, we intervene, to try and prevent falls as much as possible.*

3.3 Post-fall management element

All stakeholders ranked the post-fall management element as their third priority. They did not provide a lot of depth concerning this element, claiming that post-fall management is a standard procedure that must be carried out every time an older person falls.

M1: *...obviously, post-fall management is important. You need a good system in place to work efficiently and try to prevent errors as much as possible.*

The post-fall management element comprised two categories: procedural and participatory. The stakeholders had different opinions. The RP ranked the procedural category as the top priority placing the participatory category in the second rank. The RP clarified that the nursing staff should prioritise the care of the resident older person if an urgent matter occurs. From the regulator's point of view, documentation (a component of the procedural category) of falls is of the highest importance.

RP: *I think both [procedural and participatory] are important. But I always emphasise on documentation and reporting of falls. So I would choose this [procedural].*

On the other hand, both the organisational and operational levels agreed that the participatory and procedural categories should be considered equally important. They all agreed that every case is different. However, both categories should be carried out simultaneously. The healthcare professionals at the operational level added that documentation could inform the intervention. FG 2 discussed how certain documentation could inform healthcare professionals on what is particularly needed for the older person.

FG 1 Nurse 1: *I think they should both be on the same level. They always happen simultaneously.*

FG 1 Nurse 2: *And generally, the incident report guides us to who we are going to refer. So, they are related with each other.*

In contrast, the participant older persons had a different perspective, and prioritised the participatory category over the procedural. They all considered that having direct care is more important than documentation, although they still acknowledged that documentation is essential.

POP 2: *This [participatory] is more important than writing up in the file. However, it's still important to report everything.*

An additional point brought up by the RP, care home managers and healthcare professionals was the importance of the involvement of legal responsible persons or relatives. The stakeholders considered that the support and cooperation of legal responsible persons are crucial, especially by providing mobility aids and footwear. Moreover, consulting with the legal responsible person maintains trust and collaboration. This component was not included in the evaluated conceptual framework and this component was added to the evidence-based consolidated falls management framework, under the participatory category.

M2: *...inform the relatives [legal responsible person]! It's very important to keep them in the loop of everything. And if you refrain from informing the relatives [legal responsible person], it can lead to negative consequences because they tend to think that we [organisational and operational level employees] are trying to hide something... you'll lose their trust...*

3.4 Regulatory and organisational levels as elements

The regulatory, organisational and operational level stakeholders agreed that the regulatory and organisational levels should not be considered as stand-alone elements but should be included as members of the falls management team. The implementation of policies, regulatory standards auditing, and environmental modifications all lie under the responsibility of regulation and organisational levels and are key stakeholders of falls management.

FG 2: *They [organisation and regulation] are part of the framework... But they contribute in every section of it. So here [referring to predictive], both of them contribute just like the nurses, or the Ots [occupational therapists]. But in a different way. So we are having different levels of care, all working together to promote patient [older person] safety. They can contribute to each theme [element] here.*

The participant older persons were not able to understand how regulation can be relevant to falls management. Some participants (POP 1 and POP 4) agreed that the involvement of organisational level stakeholders is relevant to falls management. Thus, regulatory level involvement was removed, and the organisational element was retained in the consolidated framework for participant older persons.

POP 1: *The manager is in charge of everything. He guides the nurses. Or fixes things as we discussed earlier, like tiles.*

4. Applying the evidence to build an evidence-based falls management framework for Malta

In line with the model by Barends and Rousseau (**Figure 2**) [42] evidence. From the different players was aggregated and applied to develop an evidence-based national falls management framework for older persons living in Maltese residential care home settings. This framework was developed using evidence gathered from scientific literature, from the players at regulatory, organisational and operational levels of a residential care home system, with a particular focus on the older persons themselves as primary stakeholders. In instances where players did not reach a consensus, their perspectives were compared with existing literature to ensure a comprehensive approach. All components of the consolidated framework for falls management in Malta were presented in **Figure 4**. The elements which were added on the evaluated conceptual framework (**Figure 3**) were marked with a dotted red border.

The predictive element was ranked first, followed by the preventative element and finally, the post-fall management element. The predictive element took priority since the regulatory, organisational, and operational levels agreed regarding this prioritisation. Moreover, their perspective aligns with vast literature available emphasising the importance of determining the risk of falls [10, 31, 54, 57], whereby preventative measures should be based on the predictive assessment.

The elements of regulatory and organisational-level involvement were presented horizontally across the other elements, representing that regulatory and organisational-level actors are involved across falls management. The stakeholders' perspectives align with current literature, where multiple authors consider regulatory and organisational-level actors are core team members to manage falls [10, 58–60]. Tricco et al. [60] considered that regulation was a quality indicator to improve falls management and determined that when clinical performance was audited, better service was observed, leading to better management.

Seppala and Van Der Velde [31] stated that organisational-level service providers should ensure that older persons are provided with good quality care that follows the minimum standards. This is promoted by allocating adequate resources, providing a safe physical environment and regular staff training to provide good quality care.

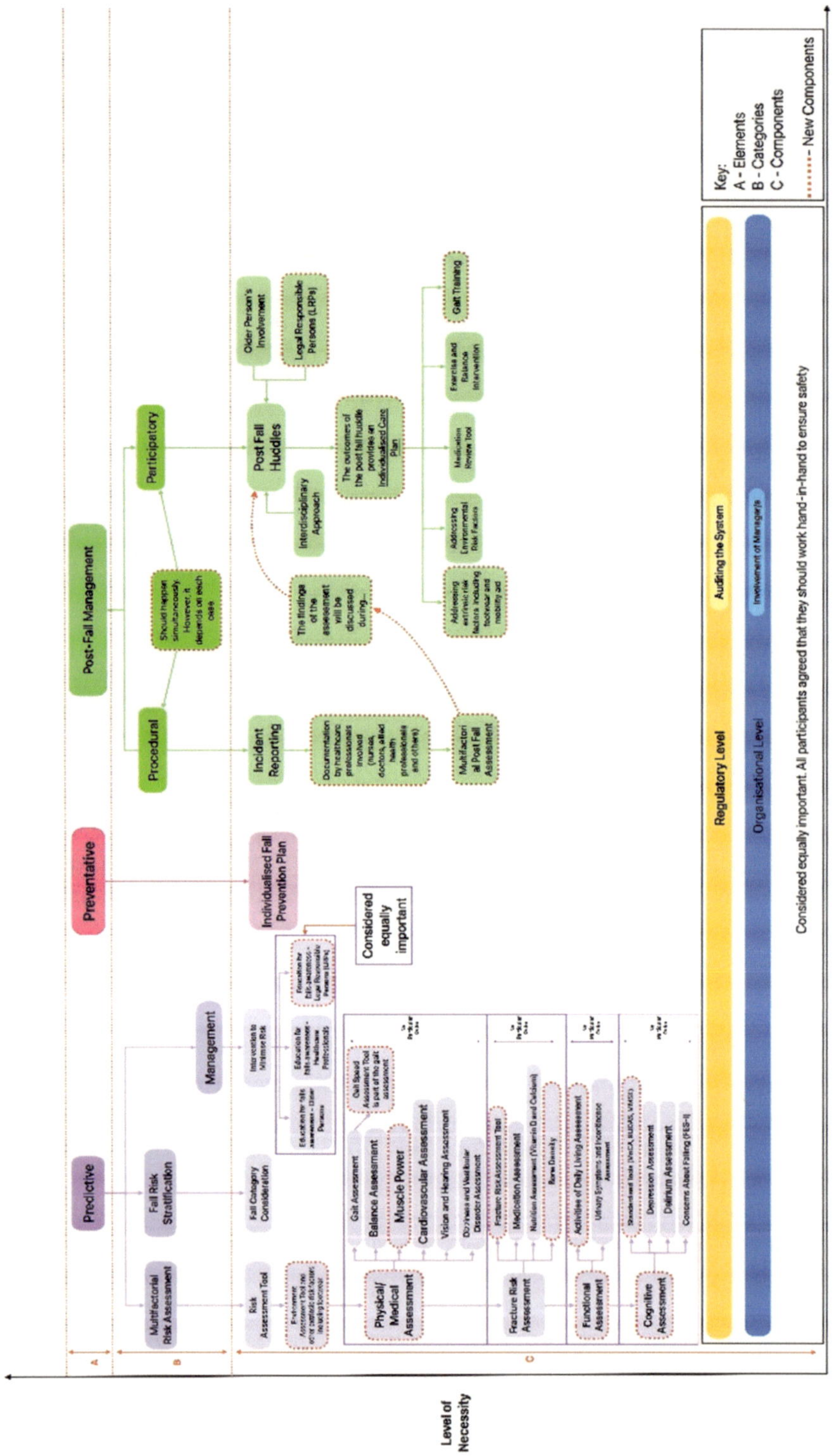

Figure 4.
The framework for falls management in malta.

The multifactorial risk assessment and fall risk stratification categories were ranked on the same level, followed by the management category. This aligns with Beck Jepsen et al. [54], Jehu et al. [61], and Ren and Peng [62] all of which stated that although there is no official consensus on falls management, many available guidelines emphasise the importance of conducting a comprehensive multifactorial assessment for all older persons, regardless of the setting. A multifactorial risk assessment should guide healthcare professional to target the indicated intervention to address the identified issue [31, 57, 58, 63].

Not all participant older persons were aware of fall risk stratification. As defined by the National Association Community Health Centres [64], fall risk stratification categorises older persons into low, medium, and high-risk groups, based on their risk of falls. This stratification is important for guiding service providers on the necessary interventions, tailored to each risk profile [64]. Despite this categorisation, it is crucial to note that all older persons should receive falls management intervention, regardless of their assessed risk level [10].

A critical aspect of a falls risk assessment is the use of evidence-based standardised tools. This was endorsed by the regulatory, organisational, and operational levels, who ranked this component as their priority. In Malta, the stakeholders use the Peninsula Health Falls Assessment Tool (PH-FRAT). This tool is used on admission, periodically and whenever indicated. However, this tool is not very sensitive and provides poor predictive value [65]. The Gait Speed Assessment Tool is considered as a significantly superior tool to predict falls when compared to the Timed Up and Go Test, Tandem Gait and Chair Stand Test, Berg Balance Scale, Dual Task Assessment, Single Leg Stance, and Functional Reach Test [54]. The Gait Speed Assessment Tool was presented in the evaluated conceptual falls management framework; however, the participants did not discuss its relevance in depth.

All participants agreed that the provision of education and increasing awareness of stakeholders at all system levels, including the legal responsible persons, is important. It was clear that some participant older persons had poor awareness regarding prediction of falls, fall risk stratification and regulation. The stakeholders' perspectives were aligned with those of Montero Odasso et al. [10], who recommended that a multifaceted falls management awareness programme, which should be provided to all residential care home staff and older persons. The authors emphasised that an educational component should be tailor-made, depending on the profession and the fall risk category. There was alignment between the results from the study and literature [10] on the recommendation to provide an educational component to legal responsible persons to promote awareness. The literature showed that an educational component, as part of a multifaceted falls management intervention, improved mobility, balance and reduce prevalence of falls [66]. Schoberer et al. [67] added that providing an educational component helped to empower older persons and increased their self-efficacy. In their global report, WHO [68] considered 'raising awareness' as the first pillar for fall prevention. Awareness should be provided to older persons and healthcare professionals. However, they added that the government should also provide awareness to allocate adequate resources to address this global concern [68].

The participant older persons considered the preventative element as their priority. Falls have a severe impact on physical and mental well-being [69]. Vaishya and Vaish [69] referred to this as post-fall syndrome, which reflects the psychological and emotional trauma triggered by frequent falls. This fear could lead to immobility syndrome, where the older person refrains from mobilisation to prevent falls [70].

Furthermore, some participants were admitted to a residential care home due to frequent falls. McKay et al. [71] stated that a fall, regardless of fall related injuries, is a high-risk factor for residential care home admission. Blain et al. [72] agreed and added that falls are the leading cause of admissions to a residential care home setting. These studies support the previously mentioned claim that falls are a major concern [54, 57, 73]. The concern extends beyond the prevalence and related injuries to include the significant life change of residential care home admission, which can also impact an older person's mental wellbeing and quality of life [74]. The participant older persons, two of whom were admitted due to falls, were aware of this. Thus, these negative experiences could have influenced their prioritisation of prevention since they are keen to avoid another fall at all costs.

The difference in perspectives between stakeholders seen in this study aligns well with the findings from Montero-Odasso et al. [10] and Dabkowski et al. [75] who found that the older persons were not on the same wavelength as the clinicians and emphasised that older persons and healthcare professionals should communicate and work as a team so that both parties gain insight into each other's perspectives [75]. The most important conclusion from this is that stakeholders should consider the perspectives of each other. The service provider should understand, learn, and empathise with the older persons' prioritisation of preventative measures and actions, and should consider this when considering cost and resource requirements for the implementation of preventative measures. In parallel, older persons should be made aware of the concept of prediction of falls and why it is an essential element to prevent falls.

As presented in **Figure 4**, the procedural and participatory categories of post-fall management elements were also ranked as the same priority. The results obtained from the participants at the operational level were in line with the findings from Montero-Odasso et al. [10] who recommended that both procedural and participatory categories are important, especially regarding medication review. Duffy [58] also discussed how documentation, a component of the procedural category, is a key evidence-based intervention that has reduced falls. However, Duffy [58] explained that positive results were identified when procedural components were combined with participatory components. Duffy, [58] and Montero-Odasso et al. [10] also explained that both categories inform each other since the incident reports and documentation can guide the service provider in safely managing and preventing future falls. Thus, the procedural and participatory categories were ranked on the same level on the consolidated falls management framework.

The regulatory, organisational, and operational level stakeholders also agreed that the involvement of legal responsible persons (LRPs) is an essential component and should be included under the participatory category. They emphasised that cooperation and inclusion of LRPs are vital in falls management. The stakeholders also noted that poor cooperation from legal responsible persons can affect the quality of care provided, viewing this as a barrier to implementing falls management in a residential care home setting. The National Council on Ageing [76] emphasised that LRPs should be part of the falls management team as they know the older person well and can detect specific changes, especially regarding mobility and eyesight. Thus, their input and perspective are considered very important. Montero-Odasso et al. [10] similarly remarked that a specific educational component should be provided to LRPs regarding falls management to raise awareness and improve cooperation. The education component for legal responsible persons component was added to the management category. The Agency for Healthcare Research and Quality [77] agreed that LRP engagement is essential for quality and safety improvement. In view of this, the agency encourages service providers to engage and improve communication with LRPs and inform them of changes in care or adverse events. These recommendations can improve trust and compliance [77]. LRP involvement was ranked at the same level as providing awareness to older persons and healthcare professionals.

5. Conclusion and recommendations

This study developed a framework for the management of falls in residential care home settings in Malta. Having a multifactorial and holistic falls management framework which is strategically implemented, can be effective. The development of the falls management framework was based on different sources of evidence, mainly the current literature and the players of such a framework. The building of the framework involved a collaborative approach across the system levels for residential care homes in Malta. The development of this framework included the perspective of the different stakeholders. The involvement of the regulator, the operational and the organisation levels should help to achieve alignment and collaboration between these levels towards a shared objective. Involvement of the stakeholders from the design stage helps increase stakeholder participation and collaboration during implementation. The inclusion of older persons living in a residential care home setting supports person-centered care, where the perspectives and needs of the older person are acknowledged and respected during policymaking and implementation. The falls management framework developed by this study should be formalised and adopted in the Maltese residential care home system. This should support the implementation of falls management initiatives and support a system of continuous improvement for falls management.

This study demonstrated the benefit of using evidence-based approach for the setting of a national framework across a specific healthcare system, and this principle should be maintained for the rest of this project and for the development of other policies and other frameworks. Hopefully, this framework will be effective in decreasing the rate of falls, recurrent falls, and fall-related injuries in the residential care home setting in Malta. Thus, the older person's well-being and quality of life are protected and improved.

Acknowledgements

The authors extend their sincere gratitude to all participants who contributed to the study, with special appreciation to the older persons, whose insights were invaluable. Furthermore, acknowledgement is given to Active Ageing and Community Care, as well as the Older Person Standards Authority, for their support and collaboration throughout the research process.

Conflict of interest

The authors declare no conflict of interest.

Author details

Matthew Cini[1,2]*, Ingrid Flores[2] and Patricia Vella Bonanno[3,4]

1 Department of Gerontology and Dementia Studies, Faculty for Social Wellbeing, University of Malta, Malta

2 Active Ageing Community Care, Ministry for Health and Active Ageing, Malta

3 Department of Health Systems Management and Leadership, Faculty of Health Sciences, University of Malta, Glasgow, UK

4 Strathclyde Institute of Pharmacy and Biomedical Science, University of Strathclyde, Glasgow, UK

*Address all correspondence to: matthew.cini@gov.mt

References

[1] World Health Organization. Falls. 2021. Available from: https://www.who.int/news-room/fact-sheets/detail/falls

[2] Cuevas-Trisan R. Balance problems and fall risks in the elderly. Promoting Health and Wellness in the Geriatric Patient. 2019;**35**(2):173-183

[3] Jung D, Shin S, Kim H. A fall prevention guideline for older adults living in long-term care facilities. International Nursing Review. 2014;**61**(4):525-533

[4] Datta A, Datta R, Elkins J. What factors predict falls in older adults living in nursing homes: A pilot study. Journal of Functional Morphology and Kinesiology. 2018;**4**(1):3

[5] Khow KS, Visvanathan R. Falls in the aging population. Clinics in Geriatric Medicine. 2017;**33**(3):357-368

[6] Schoene D, Heller C, Aung YN, Sieber CC, Kemmler W, Freiberger E. A systematic review on the influence of fear of falling on quality of life in older people: Is there a role for falls? Clinical Interventions in Ageing. 2019;**14**:701-719

[7] Sedlock J, Green J, Diegel-Vacek L. Geriatric fracture programs: Implementation of a geriatric fracture program. Orthopaedic Nursing. 2020;**39**(3):165-168

[8] Panneman M, Sterke CS, Eilering MJ, Blatter BM, Polinder S, Van Beeck EF. Costs and benefits of multifactorial falls prevention in nursing homes in the Netherlands. Experimental Gerontology. 2021;**143**:111173

[9] Jones KJ, Crowe J, Allen JA, Skinner AM, High R, Kennel V, et al. The impact of post-fall huddles on repeat fall rates and perceptions of safety culture: A quasi-experimental evaluation of a patient safety demonstration project. 2019;**19**(1):1-14

[10] Montero-Odasso M, van der Velde N, Martin FC, Petrovic M, Tan MP, Ryg J, et al. World guidelines for falls prevention and management for older adults: A global initiative. Age and Ageing. 2022;**51**(9):afac205

[11] Carayon P. Handbook of Human Factors and Ergonomics in Health Care and Patient Safety. 2nd ed. Boca Raton: CRC Press; 2016. ISBN: 978-1-4398-3033-8

[12] Beirão G, Patrício L, Fisk RP. Value cocreation in service ecosystems: Investigating health care at the micro, meso, and macro levels. Journal of Service Management. 2017;**28**(2):227-249

[13] Laihonen H. Knowledge structures of a health ecosystem. Journal of Health Organization and Management. 2012;**26**(4):542-558

[14] World Health Organization. The World Health Report. 2000. Available from: https://cdn.who.int/media/docs/default-source/health-financing/whr-2000.pdf?sfvrsn=95d8b803_1&download=true2023

[15] Piggott J, Woodland A. Handbook of the Economics of Population Aging. Amsterdam: Elsevier; 2016

[16] Michalos AC. Encyclopedia of Quality of Life and Well-Being Research. Netherlands Dordrecht: Springer; 2014

[17] Reibling N, Ariaans M, Wendt C. Worlds of healthcare: A healthcare

system typology of OECD countries. Health Policy. 2019;**123**(7):611-620

[18] Organisation for Economic Co-operation and Development. Tackling Wasteful Spending on Health. 2017. Available from: https://www.researchgate.net/profile/Luc-Hagenaars/publication/321107720_Tackling_Wasteful_Spending_on_HealthOECD_2017/links/5a114245a6fdccc2d799a8d9/Tackling-Wasteful-Spending-on-HealthOECD-2017.pdf#page=231

[19] Gulka HJ, Patel V, Arora T, McArthur C, Iaboni A. Efficacy and generalizability of falls prevention interventions in nursing homes: A systematic review and meta-analysis. Journal of the American Medical Directors Association. 2020;**21**(8):1024-1035. e4

[20] Sawatzky R, Kwon J-Y, Barclay R, Chauhan C, Frank L, van den Hout WB, et al. Implications of response shift for micro-, meso-, and macro-level healthcare decision-making using results of patient-reported outcome measures. Quality of Life Research. 2021;**30**:1-15

[21] Busse R, Klazinga N, Panteli D, Quentin W, Organization, W.H. Improving Healthcare Quality in Europe: Characteristics, Effectiveness and Implementation of Different Strategies. Copenhagen: World Health Organization. Regional Office for Europe; 2019

[22] Ciasullo MV, Silvia C, Palumbo R, Alessandra S. Value co-creation in the health service ecosystems: The enabling role of institutional arrangements. International Business Research. 2017;**10**(12):222-238

[23] Øyri SF, Wiig S. Linking resilience and regulation across system levels in healthcare–a multilevel study. Health Services Research. 2022;**22**(1):510

[24] Cummins, F. 2017. Chapter 4 – Business Rules. Available from: https://www.sciencedirect.com/topics/computer-science/government-regulation

[25] Fulop NJ, Ramsay AI. How organisations contribute to improving the quality of healthcare. BMJ. 2019;**365**:1-6

[26] Ministry for Active Ageing. Ministry for Active Ageing. 2022. Available from: https://mfaa.gov.mt/departments-and-bodies/?lang=en

[27] Independent. PPP for Residential Home for the Elderly. 2007. Available from: https://www.independent.com.mt/articles/2007-04-13/local-news/PPP-For-residential-home-for-the-elderly-171878

[28] Active Ageing and Community Care, (AACC). Residential Care – Active Ageing. 2021. Available from: https://aacc.gov.mt/residential-care/?lang=en

[29] Government of Malta. Older Persons Standards Authority. 2024. Available from: https://activeageing.gov.mt/public-bodies/older-persons-standards-authority/

[30] National Institute for Health and Care Excellence and C. Falls in Older People – Quality Standards. 2017. Available from: https://www.nice.org.uk/guidance/qs86/resources

[31] Seppala LJ, van der Velde N. How to tackle the global challenge of falls? Age and Ageing. 2022;**51**(11):afac264

[32] Harper S. The COVID-19 pandemic and older adults: Institutionalised ageism or pragmatic policy? Journal of Population Ageing. 2020;**13**(4):419-425

[33] Lin J. Heterogeneity in Health and Ageing. 2019. Available from: https://criticalgerontology.com/heterogeneity-health-aging/2022

[34] Jia H, Lubetkin EI, DeMichele K, Stark DS, Zack MM, Thompson WW. Prevalence, risk factors, and burden of disease for falls and balance or walking problems among older adults in the US. Preventative Medicine. 2019;**126**:105737

[35] Davis JC, Robertson MC, Ashe MC, Liu-Ambrose T, Khan KM, Marra CA. Does a home-based strength and balance programme in people aged≥ 80 years provide the best value for money to prevent falls? A systematic review of economic evaluations of falls prevention interventions. British Journal of Sports Medicine. 2010;**44**(2):80-89

[36] Health Service Executive. Service User Falls: A Practical Guide for Review. 2018. Available from: https://www.hse.ie/eng/about/who/nqpsd/qps-incident-management/incident-management/service-user-falls-a-practical-guide-for-review.pdf

[37] International Affairs and Best Practice Guidelines. Preventing Falls and Reducing Injury from Falls. 2017. Available from: https://rnao.ca/bpg/guidelines/prevention-falls-and-fall-injuries

[38] Missouri Hospital Association. Falls Prevention Toolkit. 2014. Available from: https://web.mhanet.com

[39] Stavropoulou C, Doherty C, Tosey P. How effective are incident-reporting systems for improving patient safety? A systematic literature review. The Milbank Quarterly. 2015;**93**(4):826-866

[40] Debra Wantz D, Patricia Campbell M, Dawn Troutman B, Crystal Muthler B. Contributing to a quality patient experience: Applying evidence based practice to support changes in nursing dress code policies. The Online Journal of Issues in Nursing. 2016;**21**(1):A1

[41] Connor L, Dean J, McNett M, Tydings DM, Shrout A, Gorsuch PF, et al. Evidence-based practice improves patient outcomes and healthcare system return on investment: Findings from a scoping review. 2023;**20**(1):6-15

[42] Barends E, Rousseau DM. Evidence-Based Management: How to Use Evidence to Make better Organizational Decisions. London: Kogan Page Publishers; 2018

[43] Centre for Evidence-Based Management. Critically Appraised Topics in Management and Organizations. 2017. Available from: https://cebma.org/wp-content/uploads/CEBMa-CAT-Guidelines-vs-2.0.pdf

[44] Callander J, Anstey AV, Ingram JR, Limpens J, Flohr C, Spuls PI. How to write a critically appraised topic: Evidence to underpin routine clinical practice. British Journal of Dermatology. 2017;**177**(4):1007-1013

[45] Victoria State Government: Department of Health and Human Services. Falls: Standardised Care Process. 2022. Available from: https://www.health.vic.gov.au/sites/default/files/2022-12/standardise-care-falls.PDF

[46] National Health Service. Procedure for the Prevention and Management of Adult Inpatients Falling in Hospital Settings. 2021. Available from: https://policyonline.nhslothian.scot/wp-content/uploads/2023/03/Falls%20Prevention%20Management%20for%20Adult%20Inpatients%20Procedure.pdf

[47] The Canadian Patient Safety Institute. Reducing Falls and Injuries

from Falls. 2019. Available from: https://gerascentre.com/wp-content/uploads/Reducing-Falls.pdf

[48] Department of Health Government of Western Australia. Post Fall Multidisciplinary Management Guidelines for Western Australian Health Care Settings. Perth: Post Fall Working Group Western Australia; 2018

[49] National Institute for Health and Care Excellence. Falls in Older People: Assessing Risk and Prevention. 2013. Available from: https://www.nice.org.uk/guidance/cg161

[50] Agency for Healthcare Research and Quality. Preventing Falls in Hospitals: A Toolkit for Improving Quality of Care. Available from: https://www.ahrq.gov/patient-safety/settings/hospital/fall-prevention/toolkit/index.html

[51] Centre of Excellence on Mobility, Fall Prevention and Injury in Ageing. Falls and Related Injuries in Residential Care: A Framework and Toolkit for Prevention. 2010. Available from: https://www.gerascentre.ca/wp-content/uploads/2023/04/Falls-and-Related-Injuries.pdf

[52] Australian Commission on Safety and Quality in Health Care, (ACSQHC). Preventing Falls and Harm from Falls in Older People: Best Practice Guidelines for Australian Hospitals and Residential Aged Care Facilities 2008. Australian Commission on Safety and Quality in Health Care; 2009. Available from: https://search.informit.org/documentSummary;res=APO;dn=1338

[53] Kyrdalen IL, Thingstad P, Sandvik L, Ormstad H. Associations between gait speed and well-known fall risk factors among community-dwelling older adults. Physiotherapy Research International. 2019;**24**(1):e1743

[54] Beck Jepsen D, Robinson K, Ogliari G, Montero-Odasso M, Kamkar N, Ryg J, et al. Predicting falls in older adults: An umbrella review of instruments assessing gait, balance, and functional mobility. BMC Geriatrics. 2022;**22**(1):1-27

[55] Patton J, Economy P. User Story Mapping: Discover the Whole Story, Build the Right Product. Sebastopol: O'Reilly Media, Inc.; 2014

[56] Braun V, Clarke V. Thematic Analysis: A Practical Guide. 2nd ed. London: SAGE Publications; 2022. ISBN: 978-1473953246

[57] Montero-Odasso MM, Kamkar N, Pieruccini-Faria F, Osman A, Sarquis-Adamson Y, Close J, et al. Evaluation of clinical practice guidelines on fall prevention and management for older adults: A systematic review. JAMA Network Open. 2021;**4**(12):e2138911 Available from: https://jamanetwork.com/journals/jamanetworkopen/fullarticle/2787179

[58] Duffy A. The assessment and management of falls in residential care settings. British Journal of Nursing. 2013;**22**(5):259-263

[59] MacLaurin A, McConnell H. Utilizing quality improvement methods to prevent falls and injury from falls: Enhancing resident safety in long-term care. Journal of Safety Research. 2011;**42**(6):525-535

[60] Tricco AC, Thomas SM, Veroniki AA, Hamid JS, Cogo E, Strifler L, et al. Quality improvement strategies to prevent falls in older adults: A systematic review and network meta-analysis. Age and Ageing. 2019;**48**(3):337-346

[61] Jehu DA, Davis JC, Falck RS, Bennett KJ, Tai D, Souza MF, et al. Risk

factors for recurrent falls in older adults: A systematic review with meta-analysis. Maturitas. 2021;**144**:23-28

[62] Ren L, Peng Y. Research of fall detection and fall prevention technologies: A systematic review. IEEE Access. 2019;**7**:77702-77722

[63] Moncada LVV, Mire LG. Preventing falls in older persons. American Family Physician. 2017;**96**(4):240-247

[64] National Association Community Health Centres. Population Health Management: Risk Stratification. 2019. Available from: https://www.nachc.org/wp-content/uploads/2019/03/Risk-Stratification-Action-Guide-Mar-2019.pdf

[65] Wabe N, Siette J, Seaman KL, Nguyen AD, Raban MZ, Close JC, et al. The use and predictive performance of the peninsula health falls risk assessment tool (PH-FRAT) in 25 residential aged care facilities: A retrospective cohort study using routinely collected data. BMC Geriatrics. 2022;**22**(1):271

[66] Najafi-Ghezeljeh T, Ghasemifard F, Jafari-Oori M. The effects of a multicomponent fall prevention intervention on fall prevalence, depression, and balance among nursing home residents. Nursing and Midwifery Studyes. 2019;**2**:78-84

[67] Schoberer D, Leino-Kilpi H, Breimaier HE, Halfens RJ, Lohrmann C. Educational interventions to empower nursing home residents: A systematic literature review. Clinical Interventions in Ageing. 2016;**11**:1351-1363

[68] World Health Organization. WHO Global Report on Falls Prevention in Older Age. Geneva: World Health Organization; 2008

[69] Vaishya R, Vaish A. Falls in older adults are serious. Indian Journal of Orthopaedics. 2020;**54**:69-74

[70] Ganji R. Empowering elderly patients to overcome "self-imposed immobility" due to fear of falling. Honk Kong Medical Journal. 2018;**24**(6):643-642

[71] McKay MA, Todd-Magel C, Copel L. Factors associated with the risk for falls in PACE participants. Geriatric Nursing. 2020;**41**(5):571-578

[72] Blain H, Miot S, Bernard PL. How Can we Prevent Falls? Cham: Springer International Publishing; 2021

[73] Montero-Odasso M, Van Der Velde N, Alexander NB, Becker C, Blain H, Camicioli R, et al. New horizons in falls prevention and management for older adults: A global initiative. Age and Ageing. 2021;**50**(5):1499-1507

[74] Bom J, Bakx P, Rellstab S. Well-being right before and after a permanent nursing home admission. 2022;**31**(12):2558-2574

[75] Dabkowski E, Cooper S, Duncan JR, Missen K. Adult inpatients' perceptions of their fall risk: A scoping review. In: Healthcare. Basel: MDPI; 2022. p. 995

[76] National Council on Ageing. Family Caregivers: Part of the Falls Prevention Team. 2019. Available from: https://www.ncoa.org/article/family-caregivers-part-of-the-falls-prevention-team

[77] Agency for Healthcare Research and Quality. Guide to Patient and Family Engagement in Hospital Quality and Safety. 2023. Available from: https://www.ahrq.gov/patient-safety/patients-families/engagingfamilies/index.html